# THIS CYCLING LOG BOOK

## BELONGS TO:
_____

# DEDICATION

This Cycling Notebook is dedicated to all the Cyclists out there who love to plan out and track hours of bike riding, and document their findings in the process.

You are my inspiration for producing books and I'm honored to be a part of keeping all of your cycling information and records organized.

# How to use this Cycling Log Book:

This useful cycling log book is a must-have for anyone that needs to record their bike riding adventures! You will love this easy to use journal to track and record all your cycling activities.

Each interior page includes space to record & track the following:

1. Date - Write down the date the start date of the cycling practice or competition.
2. Route - Use this space to fill in the location of the cycling event.
3. Distance/Duration - Record the distance of your bike ride.
4. Weather Conditions - Fill in the space from sunny to snowy weather. Write in the temperature of the day.
5. Bike Set Up - Stay on task by filling in your bicycle type, equipment and any extras for this ride.
6. Route Highlights - Record any milestones, stops along the way, time, distance and any additional notes.
7. Environment - Write down any plants or animals along the route.
8. Route Rating - From 1-5 rating, use the stars to check mark the difficulty, road conditions, and environment of the bike ride route.

If you are new to the world of cycling or have been at it for a while, this cycling log book is a must have! Can make a great useful gift for anyone that loves a good bike riding adventure!

Have Fun!

| | |
|---|---|
| 📅 DATE | |
| 🕐 TIME | |
| 🗺️ ROUTE | |

## WEATHER CONDITIONS

🌡️ _____  ☀️  ⛅  🌧️  ⛈️  ❄️
🚩 _____  ☐   ☐   ☐   ☐   ☐

| | |
|---|---|
| 📍 DISTANCE | |
| ⏱️ DURATION | |
| 🎚️ AVG SPEED | |
| 🚲 MAX SPEED | |
| ⛰️ ELEVATION GAIN | |

## BIKE SET-UP

| | |
|---|---|
| 🚲 BICYCLE TYPE | |
| 🎒 EQUIPMENT & EXTRAS | |

## ROUTE HIGHLIGHTS

| 🚩 MILESTONES & STOPS | 📍 TIME & DISTANCE | 📝 NOTES |
|---|---|---|
| | | |
| | | |
| | | |
| | | |
| | | |

## ENVIRONMENT

| | |
|---|---|
| 🌳 PLANTS | |
| | |
| | |
| 🦆 ANIMALS | |
| | |
| | |

## ROUTE RATING

| | | |
|---|---|---|
| 🏆 DIFFICULTY | | ☆☆☆☆☆ |
| 🛣️ ROAD CONDITION | | ☆☆☆☆☆ |
| 🏞️ ENVIRONMENT | | ☆☆☆☆☆ |

### ADDITIONAL NOTES

| DATE |  |
|---|---|
| TIME |  |
| ROUTE |  |

## WEATHER CONDITIONS

🌡 _____  ☀ ⛅ 🌧 ⛈ ❄
🚩 _____  ☐ ☐ ☐ ☐ ☐

| DISTANCE |  |
|---|---|
| DURATION |  |
| AVG SPEED |  |
| MAX SPEED |  |
| ELEVATION GAIN |  |

## BIKE SET-UP

| BICYCLE TYPE |  |
|---|---|
| EQUIPMENT & EXTRAS |  |

## ROUTE HIGHLIGHTS

| MILESTONES & STOPS | TIME & DISTANCE | NOTES |
|---|---|---|
|  |  |  |
|  |  |  |
|  |  |  |
|  |  |  |
|  |  |  |

## ENVIRONMENT

| PLANTS |  |
|---|---|
| ANIMALS |  |

## ROUTE RATING

| DIFFICULTY | ☆☆☆☆☆ |
|---|---|
| ROAD CONDITION | ☆☆☆☆☆ |
| ENVIRONMENT | ☆☆☆☆☆ |

### ADDITIONAL NOTES

|  | DATE |
|---|---|
|  | TIME |
|  | ROUTE |

### WEATHER CONDITIONS

| 🌡️ | ___ | ☀️ | ⛅ | 🌧️ | ⛈️ | ❄️ |
|---|---|---|---|---|---|---|
| 🎏 | ___ | ☐ | ☐ | ☐ | ☐ | ☐ |

|  |  |
|---|---|
|  | DISTANCE |
|  | DURATION |
|  | AVG SPEED |
|  | MAX SPEED |
|  | ELEVATION GAIN |

### BIKE SET-UP

|  |  |
|---|---|
|  | BICYCLE TYPE |
|  |  |
|  | EQUIPMENT & EXTRAS |
|  |  |

### ROUTE HIGHLIGHTS

| 🚩 MILESTONES & STOPS | 📍 TIME & DISTANCE | 📝 NOTES |
|---|---|---|
|  |  |  |
|  |  |  |
|  |  |  |
|  |  |  |
|  |  |  |

### ENVIRONMENT

| PLANTS |
|---|
|  |
|  |
| ANIMALS |
|  |
|  |

### ROUTE RATING

| 🏆 DIFFICULTY | ☆☆☆☆☆ |
|---|---|
| 🛣️ ROAD CONDITION | ☆☆☆☆☆ |
| ⛰️ ENVIRONMENT | ☆☆☆☆☆ |

### ADDITIONAL NOTES

## DATE

## TIME

## ROUTE

## WEATHER CONDITIONS

☀ ⛅ 🌧 ⛈ ❄

## DISTANCE

## DURATION

## AVG SPEED

## MAX SPEED

## ELEVATION GAIN

## BIKE SET-UP

### BICYCLE TYPE

### EQUIPMENT & EXTRAS

## ROUTE HIGHLIGHTS

| MILESTONES & STOPS | TIME & DISTANCE | NOTES |
|---|---|---|
|  |  |  |
|  |  |  |
|  |  |  |
|  |  |  |
|  |  |  |

## ENVIRONMENT

### PLANTS

### ANIMALS

## ROUTE RATING

DIFFICULTY ☆☆☆☆☆

ROAD CONDITION ☆☆☆☆☆

ENVIRONMENT ☆☆☆☆☆

### ADDITIONAL NOTES

## Ride Log

**DATE**

**TIME**

**ROUTE**

**WEATHER CONDITIONS**

🌡 ____  ☀️  ⛅  🌧  ⛈  ❄️

🚩 ____  ☐  ☐  ☐  ☐  ☐

**DISTANCE**

**DURATION**

**AVG SPEED**

**MAX SPEED**

**ELEVATION GAIN**

**BIKE SET-UP**

BICYCLE TYPE

EQUIPMENT & EXTRAS

### ROUTE HIGHLIGHTS

| MILESTONES & STOPS | TIME & DISTANCE | NOTES |
|---|---|---|
|  |  |  |
|  |  |  |
|  |  |  |
|  |  |  |
|  |  |  |

### ENVIRONMENT

**PLANTS**

**ANIMALS**

### ROUTE RATING

| | | |
|---|---|---|
| 🏆 DIFFICULTY | | ☆☆☆☆☆ |
| 🛣 ROAD CONDITION | | ☆☆☆☆☆ |
| ⛰ ENVIRONMENT | | ☆☆☆☆☆ |

**ADDITIONAL NOTES**

| DATE |
|---|
| TIME |
| ROUTE |

## WEATHER CONDITIONS

🌡 ___  ☀ ⛅ 🌧 ⛈ ❄
🚩 ___  ☐ ☐ ☐ ☐ ☐

| DISTANCE |
|---|
| DURATION |
| AVG SPEED |
| MAX SPEED |
| ELEVATION GAIN |

## BIKE SET-UP

| BICYCLE TYPE |
|---|
| |
| EQUIPMENT & EXTRAS |
| |

## ROUTE HIGHLIGHTS

| MILESTONES & STOPS | TIME & DISTANCE | NOTES |
|---|---|---|
| | | |
| | | |
| | | |
| | | |
| | | |

## ENVIRONMENT

| PLANTS |
|---|
| |
| ANIMALS |
| |

## ROUTE RATING

| DIFFICULTY | ☆☆☆☆☆ |
|---|---|
| ROAD CONDITION | ☆☆☆☆☆ |
| ENVIRONMENT | ☆☆☆☆☆ |

### ADDITIONAL NOTES

| DATE |
|---|
| TIME |
| ROUTE |

| WEATHER CONDITIONS |
|---|
| 🌡 ___  ☀ ⛅ 🌧 ⛈ ❄ |
| 🚩 ___  ☐ ☐ ☐ ☐ ☐ |

| DISTANCE |
|---|
| DURATION |
| AVG SPEED |
| MAX SPEED |
| ELEVATION GAIN |

| BIKE SET-UP |
|---|
| BICYCLE TYPE |
| |
| EQUIPMENT & EXTRAS |
| |

### ROUTE HIGHLIGHTS

| MILESTONES & STOPS | TIME & DISTANCE | NOTES |
|---|---|---|
| | | |
| | | |
| | | |
| | | |
| | | |

### ENVIRONMENT

| PLANTS |
|---|
| |
| |
| ANIMALS |
| |
| |

### ROUTE RATING

| DIFFICULTY | ☆☆☆☆☆ |
|---|---|
| ROAD CONDITION | ☆☆☆☆☆ |
| ENVIRONMENT | ☆☆☆☆☆ |

| ADDITIONAL NOTES |
|---|
| |

| | DATE |
|---|---|
| | TIME |
| | ROUTE |

## WEATHER CONDITIONS

| 🌡 | — | ☀ | ⛅ | 🌧 | ⛈ | ❄ |
|---|---|---|---|---|---|---|
| 🚩 | — | ☐ | ☐ | ☐ | ☐ | ☐ |

| | DISTANCE |
|---|---|
| | DURATION |
| | AVG SPEED |
| | MAX SPEED |
| | ELEVATION GAIN |

## BIKE SET-UP

| | BICYCLE TYPE |
|---|---|
| | EQUIPMENT & EXTRAS |

## ROUTE HIGHLIGHTS

| 🚩 MILESTONES & STOPS | 📍 TIME & DISTANCE | 📝 NOTES |
|---|---|---|
| | | |
| | | |
| | | |
| | | |
| | | |

## ENVIRONMENT

| | PLANTS |
|---|---|
| | |
| | ANIMALS |
| | |

## ROUTE RATING

| | DIFFICULTY | ☆☆☆☆☆ |
|---|---|---|
| | ROAD CONDITION | ☆☆☆☆☆ |
| | ENVIRONMENT | ☆☆☆☆☆ |

### ADDITIONAL NOTES

|  | DATE |
|---|---|
|  | TIME |
|  | ROUTE |

## WEATHER CONDITIONS

🌡️ ____ ☀️ ⛅ 🌧️ ⛈️ ❄️

🚩 ____ ☐ ☐ ☐ ☐ ☐

|  | DISTANCE |
|---|---|
|  | DURATION |
|  | AVG SPEED |
|  | MAX SPEED |
|  | ELEVATION GAIN |

## BIKE SET-UP

|  | BICYCLE TYPE |
|---|---|
|  | EQUIPMENT & EXTRAS |

## ROUTE HIGHLIGHTS

| 🚩 MILESTONES & STOPS | 📍 TIME & DISTANCE | 📝 NOTES |
|---|---|---|
|  |  |  |
|  |  |  |
|  |  |  |
|  |  |  |
|  |  |  |

## ENVIRONMENT

|  | PLANTS |
|---|---|
|  |  |
|  | ANIMALS |
|  |  |

## ROUTE RATING

|  | DIFFICULTY | ☆☆☆☆☆ |
|---|---|---|
|  | ROAD CONDITION | ☆☆☆☆☆ |
|  | ENVIRONMENT | ☆☆☆☆☆ |

### ADDITIONAL NOTES

| DATE | | WEATHER CONDITIONS | |
|---|---|---|---|
| TIME | | 🌡 ___ ☀ ⛅ 🌧 ⛈ ❄ | |
| ROUTE | | 🚩 ___ ☐ ☐ ☐ ☐ ☐ | |

| DISTANCE | | BIKE SET-UP | |
|---|---|---|---|
| DURATION | | BICYCLE TYPE | |
| AVG SPEED | | | |
| MAX SPEED | | EQUIPMENT & EXTRAS | |
| ELEVATION GAIN | | | |

## ROUTE HIGHLIGHTS

| MILESTONES & STOPS | TIME & DISTANCE | NOTES |
|---|---|---|
|  |  |  |
|  |  |  |
|  |  |  |
|  |  |  |
|  |  |  |

## ENVIRONMENT

| PLANTS |
|---|
|  |
| ANIMALS |
|  |

## ROUTE RATING

| DIFFICULTY | ☆☆☆☆☆ |
|---|---|
| ROAD CONDITION | ☆☆☆☆☆ |
| ENVIRONMENT | ☆☆☆☆☆ |

### ADDITIONAL NOTES

|  | DATE |
|---|---|
|  | TIME |
|  | ROUTE |

## WEATHER CONDITIONS

| 🌡 | ___ | ☀ | ⛅ | 🌧 | ⛈ | ❄ |
|---|---|---|---|---|---|---|
| 🚩 | ___ | ☐ | ☐ | ☐ | ☐ | ☐ |

|  | DISTANCE |
|---|---|
|  | DURATION |
|  | AVG SPEED |
|  | MAX SPEED |
|  | ELEVATION GAIN |

## BIKE SET-UP

|  | BICYCLE TYPE |
|---|---|
|  |  |
|  | EQUIPMENT & EXTRAS |
|  |  |

## ROUTE HIGHLIGHTS

| 🚩 MILESTONES & STOPS | 📍 TIME & DISTANCE | 📝 NOTES |
|---|---|---|
|  |  |  |
|  |  |  |
|  |  |  |
|  |  |  |
|  |  |  |

## ENVIRONMENT

|  | PLANTS |
|---|---|
|  |  |
|  |  |
|  | ANIMALS |
|  |  |
|  |  |

## ROUTE RATING

|  | DIFFICULTY | ☆☆☆☆☆ |
|---|---|---|
|  | ROAD CONDITION | ☆☆☆☆☆ |
|  | ENVIRONMENT | ☆☆☆☆☆ |

### ADDITIONAL NOTES

| DATE |
|---|
| TIME |
| ROUTE |

| WEATHER CONDITIONS |
|---|
| 🌡 ___  ☀ ⛅ 🌧 ⛈ ❄ |
| 🚩 ___  ☐ ☐ ☐ ☐ ☐ |

| DISTANCE |
|---|
| DURATION |
| AVG SPEED |
| MAX SPEED |
| ELEVATION GAIN |

| BIKE SET-UP |
|---|
| BICYCLE TYPE |
| EQUIPMENT & EXTRAS |

## ROUTE HIGHLIGHTS

| MILESTONES & STOPS | TIME & DISTANCE | NOTES |
|---|---|---|
|  |  |  |
|  |  |  |
|  |  |  |
|  |  |  |
|  |  |  |

## ENVIRONMENT

| PLANTS |
|---|
|  |
| ANIMALS |
|  |

## ROUTE RATING

| DIFFICULTY | ☆☆☆☆☆ |
|---|---|
| ROAD CONDITION | ☆☆☆☆☆ |
| ENVIRONMENT | ☆☆☆☆☆ |

### ADDITIONAL NOTES

|  | DATE |
|---|---|
|  | TIME |
|  | ROUTE |

## WEATHER CONDITIONS

🌡 _____  ☀ ⛅ 🌧 ⛈ ❄
🪁 _____  ☐ ☐ ☐ ☐ ☐

|  | DISTANCE |
|---|---|
|  | DURATION |
|  | AVG SPEED |
|  | MAX SPEED |
|  | ELEVATION GAIN |

## BIKE SET-UP

| | BICYCLE TYPE |
|---|---|
| | EQUIPMENT & EXTRAS |

## ROUTE HIGHLIGHTS

| MILESTONES & STOPS | TIME & DISTANCE | NOTES |
|---|---|---|
| | | |
| | | |
| | | |
| | | |
| | | |

## ENVIRONMENT

| PLANTS | |
|---|---|
| | |
| ANIMALS | |
| | |

## ROUTE RATING

| DIFFICULTY | ☆☆☆☆☆ |
|---|---|
| ROAD CONDITION | ☆☆☆☆☆ |
| ENVIRONMENT | ☆☆☆☆☆ |

### ADDITIONAL NOTES

|  | DATE |
|---|---|
|  | TIME |
|  | ROUTE |

### WEATHER CONDITIONS

| 🌡 | — | ☀ | ⛅ | 🌧 | ⛈ | ❄ |
|---|---|---|---|---|---|---|
| 🚩 | — | ☐ | ☐ | ☐ | ☐ | ☐ |

|  | DISTANCE |
|---|---|
|  | DURATION |
|  | AVG SPEED |
|  | MAX SPEED |
|  | ELEVATION GAIN |

### BIKE SET-UP

|  | BICYCLE TYPE |
|---|---|
|  | |
|  | EQUIPMENT & EXTRAS |
|  | |

### ROUTE HIGHLIGHTS

| MILESTONES & STOPS | TIME & DISTANCE | NOTES |
|---|---|---|
|  |  |  |
|  |  |  |
|  |  |  |
|  |  |  |
|  |  |  |

### ENVIRONMENT

| PLANTS |
|---|
|  |
|  |
| ANIMALS |
|  |
|  |

### ROUTE RATING

| DIFFICULTY | ☆☆☆☆☆ |
|---|---|
| ROAD CONDITION | ☆☆☆☆☆ |
| ENVIRONMENT | ☆☆☆☆☆ |

#### ADDITIONAL NOTES

| DATE | |
|---|---|
| TIME | |
| ROUTE | |

| WEATHER CONDITIONS | | | | | |
|---|---|---|---|---|---|
| 🌡 ___ | ☀ | ⛅ | 🌦 | ⛈ | ❄ |
| 🚩 ___ | ☐ | ☐ | ☐ | ☐ | ☐ |

| DISTANCE | |
|---|---|
| DURATION | |
| AVG SPEED | |
| MAX SPEED | |
| ELEVATION GAIN | |

## BIKE SET-UP

| BICYCLE TYPE | |
|---|---|
| EQUIPMENT & EXTRAS | |

## ROUTE HIGHLIGHTS

| MILESTONES & STOPS | TIME & DISTANCE | NOTES |
|---|---|---|
| | | |
| | | |
| | | |
| | | |
| | | |

## ENVIRONMENT

| PLANTS | |
|---|---|
| ANIMALS | |

## ROUTE RATING

| DIFFICULTY | ☆☆☆☆☆ |
|---|---|
| ROAD CONDITION | ☆☆☆☆☆ |
| ENVIRONMENT | ☆☆☆☆☆ |

### ADDITIONAL NOTES

|  | DATE |
|--|------|
|  | TIME |
|  | ROUTE |

## WEATHER CONDITIONS

| 🌡️ | — | ☀️ | ⛅ | 🌧️ | ⛈️ | ❄️ |
|----|---|----|----|----|----|----|
| 🚩 | — | ☐ | ☐ | ☐ | ☐ | ☐ |

|  |  |
|--|--|
|  | DISTANCE |
|  | DURATION |
|  | AVG SPEED |
|  | MAX SPEED |
|  | ELEVATION GAIN |

## BIKE SET-UP

|  |  |
|--|--|
|  | BICYCLE TYPE |
|  |  |
|  | EQUIPMENT & EXTRAS |
|  |  |

## ROUTE HIGHLIGHTS

| MILESTONES & STOPS | TIME & DISTANCE | NOTES |
|--------------------|-----------------|-------|
|                    |                 |       |
|                    |                 |       |
|                    |                 |       |
|                    |                 |       |
|                    |                 |       |

## ENVIRONMENT

|  |  |
|--|--|
|  | PLANTS |
|  |  |
|  |  |
|  | ANIMALS |
|  |  |
|  |  |

## ROUTE RATING

|  |  |  |
|--|--|--|
|  | DIFFICULTY | ☆☆☆☆☆ |
|  | ROAD CONDITION | ☆☆☆☆☆ |
|  | ENVIRONMENT | ☆☆☆☆☆ |

### ADDITIONAL NOTES

| DATE |
|---|
| TIME |
| ROUTE |

## WEATHER CONDITIONS

🌡 _____ ☀ ⛅ 🌧 ⛈ ❄
🚩 _____ ☐ ☐ ☐ ☐ ☐

| DISTANCE |
|---|
| DURATION |
| AVG SPEED |
| MAX SPEED |
| ELEVATION GAIN |

## BIKE SET-UP

| BICYCLE TYPE |
|---|
| |
| EQUIPMENT & EXTRAS |
| |

## ROUTE HIGHLIGHTS

| MILESTONES & STOPS | TIME & DISTANCE | NOTES |
|---|---|---|
| | | |
| | | |
| | | |
| | | |
| | | |

## ENVIRONMENT

| PLANTS |
|---|
| |
| ANIMALS |
| |

## ROUTE RATING

| DIFFICULTY | ☆☆☆☆☆ |
|---|---|
| ROAD CONDITION | ☆☆☆☆☆ |
| ENVIRONMENT | ☆☆☆☆☆ |

### ADDITIONAL NOTES

| DATE | | WEATHER CONDITIONS | |
|---|---|---|---|
| TIME | | ☀️ ⛅ 🌧️ ⛈️ ❄️ | |
| ROUTE | | ☐ ☐ ☐ ☐ ☐ | |

| DISTANCE | | BIKE SET-UP | |
|---|---|---|---|
| DURATION | | BICYCLE TYPE | |
| AVG SPEED | | | |
| MAX SPEED | | EQUIPMENT & EXTRAS | |
| ELEVATION GAIN | | | |

## ROUTE HIGHLIGHTS

| MILESTONES & STOPS | TIME & DISTANCE | NOTES |
|---|---|---|
| | | |
| | | |
| | | |
| | | |
| | | |

## ENVIRONMENT

| PLANTS |
|---|
| |
| |
| ANIMALS |
| |
| |

## ROUTE RATING

| DIFFICULTY | ☆☆☆☆☆ |
|---|---|
| ROAD CONDITION | ☆☆☆☆☆ |
| ENVIRONMENT | ☆☆☆☆☆ |

### ADDITIONAL NOTES

| DATE |
|---|
| TIME |
| ROUTE |

| WEATHER CONDITIONS |
|---|

| DISTANCE |
|---|
| DURATION |
| AVG SPEED |
| MAX SPEED |
| ELEVATION GAIN |

| BIKE SET-UP |
|---|
| BICYCLE TYPE |
| EQUIPMENT & EXTRAS |

## ROUTE HIGHLIGHTS

| MILESTONES & STOPS | TIME & DISTANCE | NOTES |
|---|---|---|
| | | |
| | | |
| | | |
| | | |
| | | |

## ENVIRONMENT

| PLANTS |
|---|
| ANIMALS |

## ROUTE RATING

| DIFFICULTY | ☆☆☆☆☆ |
|---|---|
| ROAD CONDITION | ☆☆☆☆☆ |
| ENVIRONMENT | ☆☆☆☆☆ |

### ADDITIONAL NOTES

## DATE

## TIME

## ROUTE

## WEATHER CONDITIONS

## DISTANCE

## DURATION

## AVG SPEED

## MAX SPEED

## ELEVATION GAIN

## BIKE SET-UP

**BICYCLE TYPE**

**EQUIPMENT & EXTRAS**

## ROUTE HIGHLIGHTS

| MILESTONES & STOPS | TIME & DISTANCE | NOTES |
|---|---|---|
|  |  |  |
|  |  |  |
|  |  |  |
|  |  |  |
|  |  |  |

## ENVIRONMENT

**PLANTS**

**ANIMALS**

## ROUTE RATING

| DIFFICULTY | ☆☆☆☆☆ |
|---|---|
| ROAD CONDITION | ☆☆☆☆☆ |
| ENVIRONMENT | ☆☆☆☆☆ |

### ADDITIONAL NOTES

|  |  |
|---|---|
| 📅 DATE |  |
| 🕐 TIME |  |
| 🗺️ ROUTE |  |

## WEATHER CONDITIONS

| 🌡️ | ___ | ☀️ | ⛅ | 🌧️ | ⛈️ | ❄️ |
|---|---|---|---|---|---|---|
| 🚩 | ___ | ☐ | ☐ | ☐ | ☐ | ☐ |

|  |  |
|---|---|
| 📍 DISTANCE |  |
| ⏱️ DURATION |  |
| 🌡️ AVG SPEED |  |
| 🚜 MAX SPEED |  |
| ⛰️ ELEVATION GAIN |  |

## BIKE SET-UP

| 🚲 BICYCLE TYPE |  |
|---|---|
| 🎒 EQUIPMENT & EXTRAS |  |

## ROUTE HIGHLIGHTS

| 🚩 MILESTONES & STOPS | 📍 TIME & DISTANCE | 📋 NOTES |
|---|---|---|
|  |  |  |
|  |  |  |
|  |  |  |
|  |  |  |
|  |  |  |

## ENVIRONMENT

| 🌳 PLANTS |  |
|---|---|
| 🦆 ANIMALS |  |

## ROUTE RATING

| 🏆 DIFFICULTY | ☆☆☆☆☆ |
|---|---|
| 🛣️ ROAD CONDITION | ☆☆☆☆☆ |
| ⛰️ ENVIRONMENT | ☆☆☆☆☆ |

### ADDITIONAL NOTES

|  | DATE |
|---|---|
|  | TIME |
|  | ROUTE |

## WEATHER CONDITIONS

| 🌡 | ___ | ☀ | ⛅ | 🌧 | ⛈ | ❄ |
|---|---|---|---|---|---|---|
| 🚩 | ___ |  | ☐ | ☐ | ☐ | ☐ | ☐ |

|  |  |
|---|---|
|  | DISTANCE |
|  | DURATION |
|  | AVG SPEED |
|  | MAX SPEED |
|  | ELEVATION GAIN |

## BIKE SET-UP

|  | BICYCLE TYPE |
|---|---|
|  | EQUIPMENT & EXTRAS |

## ROUTE HIGHLIGHTS

| 🚩 MILESTONES & STOPS | 📍 TIME & DISTANCE | 📝 NOTES |
|---|---|---|
|  |  |  |
|  |  |  |
|  |  |  |
|  |  |  |
|  |  |  |

## ENVIRONMENT

|  | PLANTS |
|---|---|
|  |  |
|  | ANIMALS |
|  |  |

## ROUTE RATING

|  | DIFFICULTY | ☆☆☆☆☆ |
|---|---|---|
|  | ROAD CONDITION | ☆☆☆☆☆ |
|  | ENVIRONMENT | ☆☆☆☆☆ |

### ADDITIONAL NOTES

| | DATE |
|---|---|
| | TIME |
| | ROUTE |

## WEATHER CONDITIONS

| 🌡 | ___ | ☀ | ⛅ | 🌧 | ⛈ | ❄ |
|---|---|---|---|---|---|---|
| 🚩 | ___ | ☐ | ☐ | ☐ | ☐ | ☐ |

| | DISTANCE |
|---|---|
| | DURATION |
| | AVG SPEED |
| | MAX SPEED |
| | ELEVATION GAIN |

## BIKE SET-UP

| | BICYCLE TYPE |
|---|---|
| | EQUIPMENT & EXTRAS |

## ROUTE HIGHLIGHTS

| 🚩 MILESTONES & STOPS | 📍 TIME & DISTANCE | 📝 NOTES |
|---|---|---|
| | | |
| | | |
| | | |
| | | |
| | | |

## ENVIRONMENT

| | PLANTS |
|---|---|
| | |
| | |
| | ANIMALS |
| | |
| | |

## ROUTE RATING

| | DIFFICULTY | ☆☆☆☆☆ |
|---|---|---|
| | ROAD CONDITION | ☆☆☆☆☆ |
| | ENVIRONMENT | ☆☆☆☆☆ |

### ADDITIONAL NOTES

| | DATE |
|---|---|
| | TIME |
| | ROUTE |

| WEATHER CONDITIONS | | | | | |
|---|---|---|---|---|---|
| 🌡 ___ | ☀ | ⛅ | 🌧 | ⛈ | ❄ |
| 🎏 ___ | ☐ | ☐ | ☐ | ☐ | ☐ |

| | DISTANCE |
|---|---|
| | DURATION |
| | AVG SPEED |
| | MAX SPEED |
| | ELEVATION GAIN |

## BIKE SET-UP

| | BICYCLE TYPE |
|---|---|
| | EQUIPMENT & EXTRAS |

## ROUTE HIGHLIGHTS

| 🚩 MILESTONES & STOPS | 📍 TIME & DISTANCE | 📋 NOTES |
|---|---|---|
| | | |
| | | |
| | | |
| | | |
| | | |

## ENVIRONMENT

| | PLANTS |
|---|---|
| | |
| | |
| | ANIMALS |
| | |
| | |

## ROUTE RATING

| | DIFFICULTY | ☆☆☆☆☆ |
|---|---|---|
| | ROAD CONDITION | ☆☆☆☆☆ |
| | ENVIRONMENT | ☆☆☆☆☆ |

### ADDITIONAL NOTES

| DATE | |
|---|---|
| TIME | |
| ROUTE | |

| WEATHER CONDITIONS | | | | | |
|---|---|---|---|---|---|
| 🌡 ___ | ☀ | ⛅ | 🌧 | ⛈ | ❄ |
| 🚩 ___ | ☐ | ☐ | ☐ | ☐ | ☐ |

| DISTANCE | |
|---|---|
| DURATION | |
| AVG SPEED | |
| MAX SPEED | |
| ELEVATION GAIN | |

## BIKE SET-UP

| BICYCLE TYPE | |
|---|---|
| EQUIPMENT & EXTRAS | |

## ROUTE HIGHLIGHTS

| MILESTONES & STOPS | TIME & DISTANCE | NOTES |
|---|---|---|
|  |  |  |
|  |  |  |
|  |  |  |
|  |  |  |
|  |  |  |

## ENVIRONMENT

| PLANTS | |
|---|---|
| ANIMALS | |

## ROUTE RATING

| DIFFICULTY | ☆☆☆☆☆ |
|---|---|
| ROAD CONDITION | ☆☆☆☆☆ |
| ENVIRONMENT | ☆☆☆☆☆ |

### ADDITIONAL NOTES

|  |  |
|---|---|
| DATE |  |
| TIME |  |
| ROUTE |  |

## WEATHER CONDITIONS

🌡 _____  ☀ ⛅ 🌧 ⛈ ❄
🚩 _____  ☐ ☐ ☐ ☐ ☐

|  |  |
|---|---|
| DISTANCE |  |
| DURATION |  |
| AVG SPEED |  |
| MAX SPEED |  |
| ELEVATION GAIN |  |

## BIKE SET-UP

| BICYCLE TYPE |  |
|---|---|
| EQUIPMENT & EXTRAS |  |

## ROUTE HIGHLIGHTS

| MILESTONES & STOPS | TIME & DISTANCE | NOTES |
|---|---|---|
|  |  |  |
|  |  |  |
|  |  |  |
|  |  |  |
|  |  |  |

## ENVIRONMENT

| PLANTS |  |
|---|---|
|  |  |
| ANIMALS |  |
|  |  |

## ROUTE RATING

| DIFFICULTY | ☆☆☆☆☆ |
|---|---|
| ROAD CONDITION | ☆☆☆☆☆ |
| ENVIRONMENT | ☆☆☆☆☆ |

### ADDITIONAL NOTES

|  | DATE |
|---|---|
|  | TIME |
|  | ROUTE |

## WEATHER CONDITIONS

🌡 _____  ☀️ ⛅ 🌦 🌧 ❄️
🚩 _____  ☐ ☐ ☐ ☐ ☐

|  | DISTANCE |
|---|---|
|  | DURATION |
|  | AVG SPEED |
|  | MAX SPEED |
|  | ELEVATION GAIN |

## BIKE SET-UP

|  | BICYCLE TYPE |
|---|---|
|  | EQUIPMENT & EXTRAS |

## ROUTE HIGHLIGHTS

| MILESTONES & STOPS | TIME & DISTANCE | NOTES |
|---|---|---|
|  |  |  |
|  |  |  |
|  |  |  |
|  |  |  |
|  |  |  |

## ENVIRONMENT

|  | PLANTS |
|---|---|
|  |  |
|  | ANIMALS |
|  |  |

## ROUTE RATING

|  | DIFFICULTY | ☆☆☆☆☆ |
|---|---|---|
|  | ROAD CONDITION | ☆☆☆☆☆ |
|  | ENVIRONMENT | ☆☆☆☆☆ |

### ADDITIONAL NOTES

## DATE
## TIME
## ROUTE

## WEATHER CONDITIONS

☀️ ⛅ 🌧️ ⛈️ ❄️

## DISTANCE
## DURATION
## AVG SPEED
## MAX SPEED
## ELEVATION GAIN

## BIKE SET-UP

### BICYCLE TYPE

### EQUIPMENT & EXTRAS

## ROUTE HIGHLIGHTS

| MILESTONES & STOPS | TIME & DISTANCE | NOTES |
|---|---|---|
| | | |
| | | |
| | | |
| | | |
| | | |

## ENVIRONMENT

### PLANTS

### ANIMALS

## ROUTE RATING

| | |
|---|---|
| DIFFICULTY | ☆☆☆☆☆ |
| ROAD CONDITION | ☆☆☆☆☆ |
| ENVIRONMENT | ☆☆☆☆☆ |

### ADDITIONAL NOTES

| DATE |
|---|
| TIME |
| ROUTE |

## WEATHER CONDITIONS

🌡 ____  ☀️ ⛅ 🌧 ⛈ ❄️
🪁 ____  ☐ ☐ ☐ ☐ ☐

| DISTANCE |
|---|
| DURATION |
| AVG SPEED |
| MAX SPEED |
| ELEVATION GAIN |

## BIKE SET-UP

| BICYCLE TYPE |
|---|
| |
| EQUIPMENT & EXTRAS |
| |

## ROUTE HIGHLIGHTS

| MILESTONES & STOPS | TIME & DISTANCE | NOTES |
|---|---|---|
| | | |
| | | |
| | | |
| | | |
| | | |

## ENVIRONMENT

| PLANTS |
|---|
| |
| ANIMALS |
| |

## ROUTE RATING

| | | |
|---|---|---|
| 🏆 | DIFFICULTY | ☆☆☆☆☆ |
| 🛣 | ROAD CONDITION | ☆☆☆☆☆ |
| ⛰ | ENVIRONMENT | ☆☆☆☆☆ |

### ADDITIONAL NOTES

|  | DATE |
|---|---|
|  | TIME |
|  | ROUTE |

## WEATHER CONDITIONS

🌡 ____ ☀ ⛅ 🌧 ⛈ ❄
🚩 ____ ☐ ☐ ☐ ☐ ☐

|  | DISTANCE |
|---|---|
|  | DURATION |
|  | AVG SPEED |
|  | MAX SPEED |
|  | ELEVATION GAIN |

### BIKE SET-UP

|  | BICYCLE TYPE |
|---|---|
|  |  |
|  | EQUIPMENT & EXTRAS |
|  |  |

### ROUTE HIGHLIGHTS

| MILESTONES & STOPS | TIME & DISTANCE | NOTES |
|---|---|---|
|  |  |  |
|  |  |  |
|  |  |  |
|  |  |  |
|  |  |  |

### ENVIRONMENT

| PLANTS |
|---|
|  |
|  |
| ANIMALS |
|  |
|  |

### ROUTE RATING

| DIFFICULTY | ☆☆☆☆☆ |
|---|---|
| ROAD CONDITION | ☆☆☆☆☆ |
| ENVIRONMENT | ☆☆☆☆☆ |

### ADDITIONAL NOTES

|  | DATE |
|---|---|
|  | TIME |
|  | ROUTE |

| WEATHER CONDITIONS | | | | | |
|---|---|---|---|---|---|
| 🌡 ___ | ☀ | ⛅ | 🌧 | ⛈ | ❄ |
| 🚩 ___ | ☐ | ☐ | ☐ | ☐ | ☐ |

|  | DISTANCE |
|---|---|
|  | DURATION |
|  | AVG SPEED |
|  | MAX SPEED |
|  | ELEVATION GAIN |

| BIKE SET-UP |
|---|
| BICYCLE TYPE |
|  |
| EQUIPMENT & EXTRAS |
|  |

### ROUTE HIGHLIGHTS

| MILESTONES & STOPS | TIME & DISTANCE | NOTES |
|---|---|---|
|  |  |  |
|  |  |  |
|  |  |  |
|  |  |  |
|  |  |  |

### ENVIRONMENT

| PLANTS |
|---|
|  |
|  |
| ANIMALS |
|  |
|  |

### ROUTE RATING

| DIFFICULTY | ☆☆☆☆☆ |
|---|---|
| ROAD CONDITION | ☆☆☆☆☆ |
| ENVIRONMENT | ☆☆☆☆☆ |

| ADDITIONAL NOTES |
|---|
|  |

|  | DATE |
|---|---|
|  | TIME |
|  | ROUTE |

## WEATHER CONDITIONS

| 🌡️ | ___ | ☀️ | ⛅ | 🌧️ | ⛈️ | ❄️ |
|---|---|---|---|---|---|---|
| 🚩 | ___ |  | ☐ | ☐ | ☐ | ☐ |

|  | DISTANCE |
|---|---|
|  | DURATION |
|  | AVG SPEED |
|  | MAX SPEED |
|  | ELEVATION GAIN |

## BIKE SET-UP

|  | BICYCLE TYPE |
|---|---|
|  |  |
|  | EQUIPMENT & EXTRAS |
|  |  |

## ROUTE HIGHLIGHTS

| 🚩 MILESTONES & STOPS | 📍 TIME & DISTANCE | 📝 NOTES |
|---|---|---|
|  |  |  |
|  |  |  |
|  |  |  |
|  |  |  |
|  |  |  |

## ENVIRONMENT

|  | PLANTS |
|---|---|
|  |  |
|  |  |
|  | ANIMALS |
|  |  |
|  |  |

## ROUTE RATING

|  | DIFFICULTY | ☆☆☆☆☆ |
|---|---|---|
|  | ROAD CONDITION | ☆☆☆☆☆ |
|  | ENVIRONMENT | ☆☆☆☆☆ |

### ADDITIONAL NOTES

| | |
|---|---|
| 📅 DATE | |
| 🕐 TIME | |
| 🗺️ ROUTE | |

## WEATHER CONDITIONS

| 🌡️ | ___ | ☀️ | ⛅ | 🌧️ | ⛈️ | ❄️ |
|---|---|---|---|---|---|---|
| 🪭 | ___ | ☐ | ☐ | ☐ | ☐ | ☐ |

| | |
|---|---|
| 📍 DISTANCE | |
| ⏱️ DURATION | |
| AVG SPEED | |
| 🚜 MAX SPEED | |
| ⛰️ ELEVATION GAIN | |

## BIKE SET-UP

| | |
|---|---|
| 🚲 BICYCLE TYPE | |
| 🎒 EQUIPMENT & EXTRAS | |

## ROUTE HIGHLIGHTS

| 🚩 MILESTONES & STOPS | 📍 TIME & DISTANCE | 📋 NOTES |
|---|---|---|
| | | |
| | | |
| | | |
| | | |
| | | |

## ENVIRONMENT

| | |
|---|---|
| 🌿 PLANTS | |
| | |
| | |
| 🦆 ANIMALS | |
| | |
| | |

## ROUTE RATING

| | | |
|---|---|---|
| 🏆 | DIFFICULTY | ☆☆☆☆☆ |
| 🛣️ | ROAD CONDITION | ☆☆☆☆☆ |
| ⛰️ | ENVIRONMENT | ☆☆☆☆☆ |

### ADDITIONAL NOTES

| DATE | |
|---|---|
| TIME | |
| ROUTE | |

## WEATHER CONDITIONS

| 🌡 | ― | ☀ | ⛅ | 🌧 | ⛈ | ❄ |
|---|---|---|---|---|---|---|
| 🎏 | ― | ☐ | ☐ | ☐ | ☐ | ☐ |

| DISTANCE | |
|---|---|
| DURATION | |
| AVG SPEED | |
| MAX SPEED | |
| ELEVATION GAIN | |

## BIKE SET-UP

| BICYCLE TYPE | |
|---|---|
| EQUIPMENT & EXTRAS | |

## ROUTE HIGHLIGHTS

| MILESTONES & STOPS | TIME & DISTANCE | NOTES |
|---|---|---|
|  |  |  |
|  |  |  |
|  |  |  |
|  |  |  |
|  |  |  |

## ENVIRONMENT

| PLANTS | |
|---|---|
| ANIMALS | |

## ROUTE RATING

| DIFFICULTY | ☆☆☆☆☆ |
|---|---|
| ROAD CONDITION | ☆☆☆☆☆ |
| ENVIRONMENT | ☆☆☆☆☆ |

### ADDITIONAL NOTES

|  | DATE |
|---|---|
|  | TIME |
|  | ROUTE |

## WEATHER CONDITIONS

| 🌡️ | — | ☀️ | ⛅ | 🌧️ | ⛈️ | ❄️ |
|---|---|---|---|---|---|---|
| 🍃 | — | ☐ | ☐ | ☐ | ☐ | ☐ |

|  |  |
|---|---|
|  | DISTANCE |
|  | DURATION |
|  | AVG SPEED |
|  | MAX SPEED |
|  | ELEVATION GAIN |

## BIKE SET-UP

|  |  |
|---|---|
|  | BICYCLE TYPE |
|  | EQUIPMENT & EXTRAS |

## ROUTE HIGHLIGHTS

| MILESTONES & STOPS | TIME & DISTANCE | NOTES |
|---|---|---|
|  |  |  |
|  |  |  |
|  |  |  |
|  |  |  |
|  |  |  |

## ENVIRONMENT

|  |  |
|---|---|
|  | PLANTS |
|  |  |
|  |  |
|  | ANIMALS |
|  |  |
|  |  |

## ROUTE RATING

| DIFFICULTY | ☆☆☆☆☆ |
|---|---|
| ROAD CONDITION | ☆☆☆☆☆ |
| ENVIRONMENT | ☆☆☆☆☆ |

### ADDITIONAL NOTES

## DATE
## TIME
## ROUTE

## WEATHER CONDITIONS

## DISTANCE
## DURATION
## AVG SPEED
## MAX SPEED
## ELEVATION GAIN

## BIKE SET-UP
BICYCLE TYPE

EQUIPMENT & EXTRAS

## ROUTE HIGHLIGHTS

| MILESTONES & STOPS | TIME & DISTANCE | NOTES |
|---|---|---|
|  |  |  |
|  |  |  |
|  |  |  |
|  |  |  |
|  |  |  |

## ENVIRONMENT
PLANTS

ANIMALS

## ROUTE RATING
DIFFICULTY ☆☆☆☆☆
ROAD CONDITION ☆☆☆☆☆
ENVIRONMENT ☆☆☆☆☆

### ADDITIONAL NOTES

|  | DATE |
|---|---|
|  | TIME |
|  | ROUTE |

## WEATHER CONDITIONS

🌡 ____  ☀️  ⛅  🌧  ⛈  ❄️

🪁 ____  ☐  ☐  ☐  ☐  ☐

|  | DISTANCE |
|---|---|
|  | DURATION |
|  | AVG SPEED |
|  | MAX SPEED |
|  | ELEVATION GAIN |

### BIKE SET-UP

| | BICYCLE TYPE |
|---|---|
| | |
| | EQUIPMENT & EXTRAS |
| | |

## ROUTE HIGHLIGHTS

| MILESTONES & STOPS | TIME & DISTANCE | NOTES |
|---|---|---|
|  |  |  |
|  |  |  |
|  |  |  |
|  |  |  |
|  |  |  |

## ENVIRONMENT

| | PLANTS |
|---|---|
| | |
| | ANIMALS |
| | |

## ROUTE RATING

| | DIFFICULTY | ☆☆☆☆☆ |
|---|---|---|
| | ROAD CONDITION | ☆☆☆☆☆ |
| | ENVIRONMENT | ☆☆☆☆☆ |

### ADDITIONAL NOTES

| DATE | |
|---|---|
| TIME | |
| ROUTE | |

## WEATHER CONDITIONS

🌡 ____ ☀️ ⛅ 🌧 ⛈ ❄️
🚩 ____ ☐ ☐ ☐ ☐ ☐

| DISTANCE | |
|---|---|
| DURATION | |
| AVG SPEED | |
| MAX SPEED | |
| ELEVATION GAIN | |

## BIKE SET-UP

| BICYCLE TYPE | |
|---|---|
| EQUIPMENT & EXTRAS | |

## ROUTE HIGHLIGHTS

| MILESTONES & STOPS | TIME & DISTANCE | NOTES |
|---|---|---|
| | | |
| | | |
| | | |
| | | |
| | | |

## ENVIRONMENT

| PLANTS | |
|---|---|
| ANIMALS | |

## ROUTE RATING

| DIFFICULTY | ☆☆☆☆☆ |
|---|---|
| ROAD CONDITION | ☆☆☆☆☆ |
| ENVIRONMENT | ☆☆☆☆☆ |

### ADDITIONAL NOTES

## Ride Log

| DATE | | WEATHER CONDITIONS | |
|---|---|---|---|
| TIME | | 🌡 ___ ☀ ⛅ 🌧 ⛈ ❄ | |
| ROUTE | | 🚩 ___ ☐ ☐ ☐ ☐ ☐ | |

| DISTANCE | | BIKE SET-UP | |
|---|---|---|---|
| DURATION | | BICYCLE TYPE | |
| AVG SPEED | | | |
| MAX SPEED | | EQUIPMENT & EXTRAS | |
| ELEVATION GAIN | | | |

### ROUTE HIGHLIGHTS

| MILESTONES & STOPS | TIME & DISTANCE | NOTES |
|---|---|---|
| | | |
| | | |
| | | |
| | | |
| | | |

### ENVIRONMENT

| PLANTS | |
|---|---|
| | |
| ANIMALS | |
| | |

### ROUTE RATING

| DIFFICULTY | ☆☆☆☆☆ |
|---|---|
| ROAD CONDITION | ☆☆☆☆☆ |
| ENVIRONMENT | ☆☆☆☆☆ |

**ADDITIONAL NOTES**

|  | DATE |
|---|---|
|  | TIME |
|  | ROUTE |

## WEATHER CONDITIONS

| 🌡️ | ___ | ☀️ | ⛅ | 🌧️ | ⛈️ | ❄️ |
|---|---|---|---|---|---|---|
| 🎐 | ___ | ☐ | ☐ | ☐ | ☐ | ☐ |

|  | DISTANCE |
|---|---|
|  | DURATION |
|  | AVG SPEED |
|  | MAX SPEED |
|  | ELEVATION GAIN |

## BIKE SET-UP

|  | BICYCLE TYPE |
|---|---|
|  | EQUIPMENT & EXTRAS |

## ROUTE HIGHLIGHTS

| 🚩 MILESTONES & STOPS | 📍 TIME & DISTANCE | 📝 NOTES |
|---|---|---|
|  |  |  |
|  |  |  |
|  |  |  |
|  |  |  |
|  |  |  |

## ENVIRONMENT

|  | PLANTS |
|---|---|
|  |  |
|  | ANIMALS |
|  |  |

## ROUTE RATING

|  | DIFFICULTY | ☆☆☆☆☆ |
|---|---|---|
|  | ROAD CONDITION | ☆☆☆☆☆ |
|  | ENVIRONMENT | ☆☆☆☆☆ |

### ADDITIONAL NOTES

| DATE |
|---|
| TIME |
| ROUTE |

## WEATHER CONDITIONS

| DISTANCE |
|---|
| DURATION |
| AVG SPEED |
| MAX SPEED |
| ELEVATION GAIN |

## BIKE SET-UP

BICYCLE TYPE

EQUIPMENT & EXTRAS

## ROUTE HIGHLIGHTS

| MILESTONES & STOPS | TIME & DISTANCE | NOTES |
|---|---|---|
|  |  |  |
|  |  |  |
|  |  |  |
|  |  |  |
|  |  |  |

## ENVIRONMENT

PLANTS

ANIMALS

## ROUTE RATING

DIFFICULTY ☆☆☆☆☆

ROAD CONDITION ☆☆☆☆☆

ENVIRONMENT ☆☆☆☆☆

### ADDITIONAL NOTES

|  | DATE |
|---|---|
|  | TIME |
|  | ROUTE |

## WEATHER CONDITIONS

| 🌡 | ___ | ☀ | ⛅ | 🌧 | ⛈ | ❄ |
| 🚩 | ___ | ☐ | ☐ | ☐ | ☐ | ☐ |

|  | DISTANCE |
|---|---|
|  | DURATION |
|  | AVG SPEED |
|  | MAX SPEED |
|  | ELEVATION GAIN |

## BIKE SET-UP

|  | BICYCLE TYPE |
|---|---|
|  |  |
|  | EQUIPMENT & EXTRAS |
|  |  |

## ROUTE HIGHLIGHTS

| MILESTONES & STOPS | TIME & DISTANCE | NOTES |
|---|---|---|
|  |  |  |
|  |  |  |
|  |  |  |
|  |  |  |
|  |  |  |

## ENVIRONMENT

| PLANTS |
|---|
|  |
|  |
| ANIMALS |
|  |
|  |

## ROUTE RATING

| DIFFICULTY | ☆☆☆☆☆ |
|---|---|
| ROAD CONDITION | ☆☆☆☆☆ |
| ENVIRONMENT | ☆☆☆☆☆ |

### ADDITIONAL NOTES

|  | DATE |
|---|---|
|  | TIME |
|  | ROUTE |

## WEATHER CONDITIONS

🌡 ____ ☀ ⛅ 🌧 ⛈ ❄
🚩 ____ ☐ ☐ ☐ ☐ ☐

|  | DISTANCE |
|---|---|
|  | DURATION |
|  | AVG SPEED |
|  | MAX SPEED |
|  | ELEVATION GAIN |

## BIKE SET-UP

|  | BICYCLE TYPE |
|---|---|
|  | EQUIPMENT & EXTRAS |

## ROUTE HIGHLIGHTS

| MILESTONES & STOPS | TIME & DISTANCE | NOTES |
|---|---|---|
|  |  |  |
|  |  |  |
|  |  |  |
|  |  |  |
|  |  |  |

## ENVIRONMENT

| PLANTS |
|---|
|  |
|  |
| ANIMALS |
|  |
|  |

## ROUTE RATING

| DIFFICULTY | ☆☆☆☆☆ |
|---|---|
| ROAD CONDITION | ☆☆☆☆☆ |
| ENVIRONMENT | ☆☆☆☆☆ |

### ADDITIONAL NOTES

## DATE
## TIME
## ROUTE

## WEATHER CONDITIONS

## DISTANCE
## DURATION
## AVG SPEED
## MAX SPEED
## ELEVATION GAIN

## BIKE SET-UP
### BICYCLE TYPE
### EQUIPMENT & EXTRAS

## ROUTE HIGHLIGHTS

| MILESTONES & STOPS | TIME & DISTANCE | NOTES |
|---|---|---|
|  |  |  |
|  |  |  |
|  |  |  |
|  |  |  |
|  |  |  |

## ENVIRONMENT
### PLANTS
### ANIMALS

## ROUTE RATING
- DIFFICULTY ☆☆☆☆☆
- ROAD CONDITION ☆☆☆☆☆
- ENVIRONMENT ☆☆☆☆☆

### ADDITIONAL NOTES

|  | DATE |
|---|---|
|  | TIME |
|  | ROUTE |

### WEATHER CONDITIONS

| 🌡 | ___ | ☀ | ⛅ | 🌧 | ⛈ | ❄ |
|---|---|---|---|---|---|---|
| 🌬 | ___ | ☐ | ☐ | ☐ | ☐ | ☐ |

|  | DISTANCE |
|---|---|
|  | DURATION |
|  | AVG SPEED |
|  | MAX SPEED |
|  | ELEVATION GAIN |

### BIKE SET-UP

|  | BICYCLE TYPE |
|---|---|
|  |  |
|  | EQUIPMENT & EXTRAS |
|  |  |

### ROUTE HIGHLIGHTS

| MILESTONES & STOPS | TIME & DISTANCE | NOTES |
|---|---|---|
|  |  |  |
|  |  |  |
|  |  |  |
|  |  |  |
|  |  |  |

### ENVIRONMENT

| PLANTS |
|---|
|  |
|  |
| ANIMALS |
|  |
|  |

### ROUTE RATING

| DIFFICULTY | ☆☆☆☆☆ |
|---|---|
| ROAD CONDITION | ☆☆☆☆☆ |
| ENVIRONMENT | ☆☆☆☆☆ |

### ADDITIONAL NOTES

|  | DATE |
|---|---|
|  | TIME |
|  | ROUTE |

## WEATHER CONDITIONS

| 🌡 | ___ | ☀ | ⛅ | 🌧 | ⛈ | ❄ |
| 🚩 | ___ | ☐ | ☐ | ☐ | ☐ | ☐ |

|  | DISTANCE |
|---|---|
|  | DURATION |
|  | AVG SPEED |
|  | MAX SPEED |
|  | ELEVATION GAIN |

## BIKE SET-UP

|  | BICYCLE TYPE |
|---|---|
|  |  |
|  | EQUIPMENT & EXTRAS |
|  |  |

## ROUTE HIGHLIGHTS

| MILESTONES & STOPS | TIME & DISTANCE | NOTES |
|---|---|---|
|  |  |  |
|  |  |  |
|  |  |  |
|  |  |  |
|  |  |  |

## ENVIRONMENT

| PLANTS |
|---|
|  |
|  |
| ANIMALS |
|  |
|  |

## ROUTE RATING

| DIFFICULTY | ☆☆☆☆☆ |
|---|---|
| ROAD CONDITION | ☆☆☆☆☆ |
| ENVIRONMENT | ☆☆☆☆☆ |

### ADDITIONAL NOTES

| | DATE |
|---|---|
| | TIME |
| | ROUTE |

## WEATHER CONDITIONS

| | DISTANCE |
|---|---|
| | DURATION |
| | AVG SPEED |
| | MAX SPEED |
| | ELEVATION GAIN |

## BIKE SET-UP

| | BICYCLE TYPE |
|---|---|
| | EQUIPMENT & EXTRAS |

## ROUTE HIGHLIGHTS

| MILESTONES & STOPS | TIME & DISTANCE | NOTES |
|---|---|---|
| | | |
| | | |
| | | |
| | | |
| | | |

## ENVIRONMENT

| | PLANTS |
|---|---|
| | ANIMALS |

## ROUTE RATING

| | DIFFICULTY | ☆☆☆☆☆ |
|---|---|---|
| | ROAD CONDITION | ☆☆☆☆☆ |
| | ENVIRONMENT | ☆☆☆☆☆ |

### ADDITIONAL NOTES

| DATE |
|---|
| TIME |
| ROUTE |

## WEATHER CONDITIONS

| 🌡 | ― | ☀ | ⛅ | 🌧 | ⛈ | ❄ |
|---|---|---|---|---|---|---|
| 🚩 | ― | ☐ | ☐ | ☐ | ☐ | ☐ |

| DISTANCE |
|---|
| DURATION |
| AVG SPEED |
| MAX SPEED |
| ELEVATION GAIN |

## BIKE SET-UP

| BICYCLE TYPE |
|---|
| |
| EQUIPMENT & EXTRAS |
| |

## ROUTE HIGHLIGHTS

| MILESTONES & STOPS | TIME & DISTANCE | NOTES |
|---|---|---|
| | | |
| | | |
| | | |
| | | |
| | | |

## ENVIRONMENT

| PLANTS |
|---|
| |
| |
| ANIMALS |
| |
| |

## ROUTE RATING

| DIFFICULTY | ☆☆☆☆☆ |
|---|---|
| ROAD CONDITION | ☆☆☆☆☆ |
| ENVIRONMENT | ☆☆☆☆☆ |

### ADDITIONAL NOTES

| DATE |  |
|---|---|
| TIME |  |
| ROUTE |  |

## WEATHER CONDITIONS

| 🌡 | ___ | ☀ | ⛅ | 🌧 | ⛈ | ❄ |
|---|---|---|---|---|---|---|
| 🚩 | ___ | ☐ | ☐ | ☐ | ☐ | ☐ |

| DISTANCE |  |
|---|---|
| DURATION |  |
| AVG SPEED |  |
| MAX SPEED |  |
| ELEVATION GAIN |  |

## BIKE SET-UP

| BICYCLE TYPE |
|---|
|  |
| EQUIPMENT & EXTRAS |
|  |

## ROUTE HIGHLIGHTS

| MILESTONES & STOPS | TIME & DISTANCE | NOTES |
|---|---|---|
|  |  |  |
|  |  |  |
|  |  |  |
|  |  |  |
|  |  |  |

## ENVIRONMENT

| PLANTS |
|---|
|  |
|  |
| ANIMALS |
|  |
|  |

## ROUTE RATING

| DIFFICULTY | ☆☆☆☆☆ |
|---|---|
| ROAD CONDITION | ☆☆☆☆☆ |
| ENVIRONMENT | ☆☆☆☆☆ |

### ADDITIONAL NOTES

## DATE

## TIME

## ROUTE

## WEATHER CONDITIONS

## DISTANCE

## DURATION

## AVG SPEED

## MAX SPEED

## ELEVATION GAIN

## BIKE SET-UP

BICYCLE TYPE

EQUIPMENT & EXTRAS

## ROUTE HIGHLIGHTS

| MILESTONES & STOPS | TIME & DISTANCE | NOTES |
|---|---|---|
|  |  |  |
|  |  |  |
|  |  |  |
|  |  |  |
|  |  |  |

## ENVIRONMENT

PLANTS

ANIMALS

## ROUTE RATING

DIFFICULTY ☆☆☆☆☆

ROAD CONDITION ☆☆☆☆☆

ENVIRONMENT ☆☆☆☆☆

### ADDITIONAL NOTES

| DATE |
|---|
| TIME |
| ROUTE |

## WEATHER CONDITIONS

| 🌡️ ___ | ☀️ | ⛅ | 🌧️ | ⛈️ | ❄️ |
|---|---|---|---|---|---|
| 🚩 ___ | ☐ | ☐ | ☐ | ☐ | ☐ |

| DISTANCE |
|---|
| DURATION |
| AVG SPEED |
| MAX SPEED |
| ELEVATION GAIN |

## BIKE SET-UP

| BICYCLE TYPE |
|---|
| |
| EQUIPMENT & EXTRAS |
| |

## ROUTE HIGHLIGHTS

| MILESTONES & STOPS | TIME & DISTANCE | NOTES |
|---|---|---|
| | | |
| | | |
| | | |
| | | |
| | | |

## ENVIRONMENT

| PLANTS |
|---|
| |
| |
| ANIMALS |
| |
| |

## ROUTE RATING

| DIFFICULTY | ☆☆☆☆☆ |
|---|---|
| ROAD CONDITION | ☆☆☆☆☆ |
| ENVIRONMENT | ☆☆☆☆☆ |

### ADDITIONAL NOTES

## Ride Log

| | |
|---|---|
| DATE | |
| TIME | |
| ROUTE | |

### WEATHER CONDITIONS

🌡 _____   ☀ ☁ 🌧 ⛈ ❄
🌬 _____   ☐ ☐ ☐ ☐ ☐

| | |
|---|---|
| DISTANCE | |
| DURATION | |
| AVG SPEED | |
| MAX SPEED | |
| ELEVATION GAIN | |

### BIKE SET-UP

| | |
|---|---|
| BICYCLE TYPE | |
| EQUIPMENT & EXTRAS | |

### ROUTE HIGHLIGHTS

| MILESTONES & STOPS | TIME & DISTANCE | NOTES |
|---|---|---|
| | | |
| | | |
| | | |
| | | |
| | | |

### ENVIRONMENT

| | |
|---|---|
| PLANTS | |
| ANIMALS | |

### ROUTE RATING

| | |
|---|---|
| DIFFICULTY | ☆☆☆☆☆ |
| ROAD CONDITION | ☆☆☆☆☆ |
| ENVIRONMENT | ☆☆☆☆☆ |

**ADDITIONAL NOTES**

| DATE | | WEATHER CONDITIONS |
|---|---|---|
| TIME | | 🌡 ___  ☀ ⛅ 🌧 ⛈ ❄ |
| ROUTE | | 🚩 ___  ☐ ☐ ☐ ☐ ☐ |

| | | BIKE SET-UP |
|---|---|---|
| DISTANCE | | BICYCLE TYPE |
| DURATION | | |
| AVG SPEED | | |
| MAX SPEED | | EQUIPMENT & EXTRAS |
| ELEVATION GAIN | | |

## ROUTE HIGHLIGHTS

| MILESTONES & STOPS | TIME & DISTANCE | NOTES |
|---|---|---|
| | | |
| | | |
| | | |
| | | |
| | | |

## ENVIRONMENT

**PLANTS**

**ANIMALS**

## ROUTE RATING

| | |
|---|---|
| DIFFICULTY | ☆☆☆☆☆ |
| ROAD CONDITION | ☆☆☆☆☆ |
| ENVIRONMENT | ☆☆☆☆☆ |

**ADDITIONAL NOTES**

|  | DATE |
|---|---|
|  | TIME |
|  | ROUTE |

### WEATHER CONDITIONS

| 🌡️ | ____ | ☀️ | ⛅ | 🌧️ | ⛈️ | ❄️ |
|---|---|---|---|---|---|---|
| 🌬️ | ____ | ☐ | ☐ | ☐ | ☐ | ☐ |

|  | DISTANCE |
|---|---|
|  | DURATION |
|  | AVG SPEED |
|  | MAX SPEED |
|  | ELEVATION GAIN |

### BIKE SET-UP

|  | BICYCLE TYPE |
|---|---|
|  |  |
|  | EQUIPMENT & EXTRAS |
|  |  |

### ROUTE HIGHLIGHTS

| MILESTONES & STOPS | TIME & DISTANCE | NOTES |
|---|---|---|
|  |  |  |
|  |  |  |
|  |  |  |
|  |  |  |
|  |  |  |

### ENVIRONMENT

| PLANTS |
|---|
|  |
|  |
| ANIMALS |
|  |
|  |

### ROUTE RATING

| DIFFICULTY | ☆☆☆☆☆ |
|---|---|
| ROAD CONDITION | ☆☆☆☆☆ |
| ENVIRONMENT | ☆☆☆☆☆ |

### ADDITIONAL NOTES

| DATE |
|---|
| TIME |
| ROUTE |

## WEATHER CONDITIONS

🌡️ ____  ☀️ ⛅ 🌧️ ⛈️ ❄️
🚩 ____  ☐ ☐ ☐ ☐ ☐

| DISTANCE |
|---|
| DURATION |
| AVG SPEED |
| MAX SPEED |
| ELEVATION GAIN |

## BIKE SET-UP

| BICYCLE TYPE |
|---|
| |
| EQUIPMENT & EXTRAS |
| |

## ROUTE HIGHLIGHTS

| MILESTONES & STOPS | TIME & DISTANCE | NOTES |
|---|---|---|
| | | |
| | | |
| | | |
| | | |
| | | |

## ENVIRONMENT

| PLANTS |
|---|
| |
| |
| ANIMALS |
| |
| |

## ROUTE RATING

| DIFFICULTY | ☆☆☆☆☆ |
|---|---|
| ROAD CONDITION | ☆☆☆☆☆ |
| ENVIRONMENT | ☆☆☆☆☆ |

### ADDITIONAL NOTES

|  | DATE |
|---|---|
|  | TIME |
|  | ROUTE |

## WEATHER CONDITIONS

| 🌡 | — | ☀ | ⛅ | 🌦 | 🌧 | ❄ |
| 🚩 | — | ☐ | ☐ | ☐ | ☐ | ☐ |

|  | DISTANCE |
|---|---|
|  | DURATION |
|  | AVG SPEED |
|  | MAX SPEED |
|  | ELEVATION GAIN |

## BIKE SET-UP

|  | BICYCLE TYPE |
|---|---|
|  |  |
|  | EQUIPMENT & EXTRAS |
|  |  |

## ROUTE HIGHLIGHTS

| MILESTONES & STOPS | TIME & DISTANCE | NOTES |
|---|---|---|
|  |  |  |
|  |  |  |
|  |  |  |
|  |  |  |
|  |  |  |

## ENVIRONMENT

|  | PLANTS |
|---|---|
|  |  |
|  | ANIMALS |
|  |  |

## ROUTE RATING

|  | DIFFICULTY | ☆☆☆☆☆ |
|---|---|---|
|  | ROAD CONDITION | ☆☆☆☆☆ |
|  | ENVIRONMENT | ☆☆☆☆☆ |

### ADDITIONAL NOTES

|  | DATE |
|---|---|
|  | TIME |
|  | ROUTE |

| WEATHER CONDITIONS | | | | | |
|---|---|---|---|---|---|
| 🌡 ____ | ☀ | ⛅ | 🌧 | ⛈ | ❄ |
| 🚩 ____ | ☐ | ☐ | ☐ | ☐ | ☐ |

|  | DISTANCE |
|---|---|
|  | DURATION |
|  | AVG SPEED |
|  | MAX SPEED |
|  | ELEVATION GAIN |

| BIKE SET-UP | |
|---|---|
|  | BICYCLE TYPE |
|  |  |
|  | EQUIPMENT & EXTRAS |
|  |  |

### ROUTE HIGHLIGHTS

| MILESTONES & STOPS | TIME & DISTANCE | NOTES |
|---|---|---|
|  |  |  |
|  |  |  |
|  |  |  |
|  |  |  |
|  |  |  |

### ENVIRONMENT

|  | PLANTS |
|---|---|
|  |  |
|  |  |
|  | ANIMALS |
|  |  |
|  |  |

### ROUTE RATING

|  | DIFFICULTY | ☆☆☆☆☆ |
|---|---|---|
|  | ROAD CONDITION | ☆☆☆☆☆ |
|  | ENVIRONMENT | ☆☆☆☆☆ |

| ADDITIONAL NOTES |
|---|
|  |
|  |

|  | DATE |
|---|---|
|  | TIME |
|  | ROUTE |

## WEATHER CONDITIONS

🌡️ ———   ☀️  ⛅  🌧️  ⛈️  ❄️
🚩 ———   ☐   ☐   ☐   ☐   ☐

|  | DISTANCE |
|---|---|
|  | DURATION |
|  | AVG SPEED |
|  | MAX SPEED |
|  | ELEVATION GAIN |

## BIKE SET-UP

|  | BICYCLE TYPE |
|---|---|
|  |  |
|  | EQUIPMENT & EXTRAS |
|  |  |

## ROUTE HIGHLIGHTS

| MILESTONES & STOPS | TIME & DISTANCE | NOTES |
|---|---|---|
|  |  |  |
|  |  |  |
|  |  |  |
|  |  |  |
|  |  |  |

## ENVIRONMENT

|  | PLANTS |
|---|---|
|  |  |
|  | ANIMALS |
|  |  |

## ROUTE RATING

| | | |
|---|---|---|
|  | DIFFICULTY | ☆☆☆☆☆ |
|  | ROAD CONDITION | ☆☆☆☆☆ |
|  | ENVIRONMENT | ☆☆☆☆☆ |

### ADDITIONAL NOTES

| DATE |
|---|
| TIME |
| ROUTE |

| WEATHER CONDITIONS |
|---|
| 🌡 ___  ☀ ⛅ 🌧 ⛈ ❄ |
| 🚩 ___  ☐ ☐ ☐ ☐ ☐ |

| DISTANCE |
|---|
| DURATION |
| AVG SPEED |
| MAX SPEED |
| ELEVATION GAIN |

| BIKE SET-UP |
|---|
| BICYCLE TYPE |
| |
| EQUIPMENT & EXTRAS |
| |

## ROUTE HIGHLIGHTS

| MILESTONES & STOPS | TIME & DISTANCE | NOTES |
|---|---|---|
| | | |
| | | |
| | | |
| | | |
| | | |

## ENVIRONMENT

| PLANTS |
|---|
| |
| |
| ANIMALS |
| |
| |

## ROUTE RATING

| DIFFICULTY | ☆☆☆☆☆ |
|---|---|
| ROAD CONDITION | ☆☆☆☆☆ |
| ENVIRONMENT | ☆☆☆☆☆ |

### ADDITIONAL NOTES

| DATE | | WEATHER CONDITIONS | | | | | |
|---|---|---|---|---|---|---|---|
| TIME | | 🌡 ___ | ☀ | ⛅ | 🌧 | ⛈ | ❄ |
| ROUTE | | 🚩 ___ | ☐ | ☐ | ☐ | ☐ | ☐ |

| | | BIKE SET-UP |
|---|---|---|
| DISTANCE | | BICYCLE TYPE |
| DURATION | | |
| AVG SPEED | | |
| MAX SPEED | | EQUIPMENT & EXTRAS |
| ELEVATION GAIN | | |

## ROUTE HIGHLIGHTS

| MILESTONES & STOPS | TIME & DISTANCE | NOTES |
|---|---|---|
| | | |
| | | |
| | | |
| | | |
| | | |

| ENVIRONMENT | | ROUTE RATING | |
|---|---|---|---|
| PLANTS | | DIFFICULTY | ☆☆☆☆☆ |
| | | ROAD CONDITION | ☆☆☆☆☆ |
| | | ENVIRONMENT | ☆☆☆☆☆ |
| ANIMALS | | ADDITIONAL NOTES | |
| | | | |

| DATE |  |
|---|---|
| TIME |  |
| ROUTE |  |

## WEATHER CONDITIONS

🌡 _____   ☀️  ⛅  🌧  ⛈  ❄️

🚩 _____   ☐   ☐   ☐   ☐   ☐

| DISTANCE |  |
|---|---|
| DURATION |  |
| AVG SPEED |  |
| MAX SPEED |  |
| ELEVATION GAIN |  |

## BIKE SET-UP

| BICYCLE TYPE |
|---|
|  |
| EQUIPMENT & EXTRAS |
|  |

## ROUTE HIGHLIGHTS

| MILESTONES & STOPS | TIME & DISTANCE | NOTES |
|---|---|---|
|  |  |  |
|  |  |  |
|  |  |  |
|  |  |  |
|  |  |  |

## ENVIRONMENT

| PLANTS |
|---|
|  |
| ANIMALS |
|  |

## ROUTE RATING

| DIFFICULTY | ☆☆☆☆☆ |
|---|---|
| ROAD CONDITION | ☆☆☆☆☆ |
| ENVIRONMENT | ☆☆☆☆☆ |

### ADDITIONAL NOTES

| DATE | WEATHER CONDITIONS |
|---|---|
| TIME | 🌡 ____ ☀ ⛅ 🌧 ⛈ ❄ |
| ROUTE | 🚩 ____ ☐ ☐ ☐ ☐ ☐ |

| | |
|---|---|
| DISTANCE | **BIKE SET-UP** |
| DURATION | BICYCLE TYPE |
| AVG SPEED | |
| MAX SPEED | EQUIPMENT & EXTRAS |
| ELEVATION GAIN | |

## ROUTE HIGHLIGHTS

| MILESTONES & STOPS | TIME & DISTANCE | NOTES |
|---|---|---|
| | | |
| | | |
| | | |
| | | |
| | | |

## ENVIRONMENT

PLANTS

ANIMALS

## ROUTE RATING

| | |
|---|---|
| DIFFICULTY | ☆☆☆☆☆ |
| ROAD CONDITION | ☆☆☆☆☆ |
| ENVIRONMENT | ☆☆☆☆☆ |

### ADDITIONAL NOTES

|  | DATE |
|---|---|
|  | TIME |
|  | ROUTE |

### WEATHER CONDITIONS

🌡️ _____  ☀️  ⛅  🌧️  ⛈️  ❄️
🚩 _____  ☐  ☐  ☐  ☐  ☐

|  | DISTANCE |
|---|---|
|  | DURATION |
|  | AVG SPEED |
|  | MAX SPEED |
|  | ELEVATION GAIN |

### BIKE SET-UP

| | BICYCLE TYPE |
|---|---|
| | |
| | EQUIPMENT & EXTRAS |
| | |

### ROUTE HIGHLIGHTS

| 🚩 MILESTONES & STOPS | 📍 TIME & DISTANCE | 📝 NOTES |
|---|---|---|
| | | |
| | | |
| | | |
| | | |
| | | |

### ENVIRONMENT

| 🌳 PLANTS |
|---|
| |
| |
| 🦆 ANIMALS |
| |
| |

### ROUTE RATING

| 🏆 DIFFICULTY | ☆☆☆☆☆ |
|---|---|
| 🛣️ ROAD CONDITION | ☆☆☆☆☆ |
| ⛰️ ENVIRONMENT | ☆☆☆☆☆ |

#### ADDITIONAL NOTES

| | |
|---|---|
| 📅 DATE | |
| 🕐 TIME | |
| 🗺️ ROUTE | |

## WEATHER CONDITIONS

🌡️ _____  ☀️  ⛅  🌧️  ⛈️  ❄️

🚩 _____  ☐  ☐  ☐  ☐  ☐

| | |
|---|---|
| 📍 DISTANCE | |
| ⏱️ DURATION | |
| 🚴 AVG SPEED | |
| 🚵 MAX SPEED | |
| ⛰️ ELEVATION GAIN | |

## BIKE SET-UP

| | |
|---|---|
| 🚲 BICYCLE TYPE | |
| 🎒 EQUIPMENT & EXTRAS | |

## ROUTE HIGHLIGHTS

| 🚩 MILESTONES & STOPS | 📍 TIME & DISTANCE | 📝 NOTES |
|---|---|---|
| | | |
| | | |
| | | |
| | | |
| | | |

## ENVIRONMENT

| | |
|---|---|
| 🌳 PLANTS | |
| 🦆 ANIMALS | |

## ROUTE RATING

| | |
|---|---|
| 🏆 DIFFICULTY | ☆☆☆☆☆ |
| 🛣️ ROAD CONDITION | ☆☆☆☆☆ |
| 🏞️ ENVIRONMENT | ☆☆☆☆☆ |

### ADDITIONAL NOTES

## Ride Log

**DATE**

**TIME**

**ROUTE**

**DISTANCE**

**DURATION**

**AVG SPEED**

**MAX SPEED**

**ELEVATION GAIN**

### WEATHER CONDITIONS

🌡 ____   ☀ ⛅ 🌧 ⛈ ❄
🚩 ____   ☐ ☐ ☐ ☐ ☐

### BIKE SET-UP

BICYCLE TYPE

EQUIPMENT & EXTRAS

### ROUTE HIGHLIGHTS

| MILESTONES & STOPS | TIME & DISTANCE | NOTES |
|---|---|---|
|  |  |  |
|  |  |  |
|  |  |  |
|  |  |  |
|  |  |  |

### ENVIRONMENT

PLANTS

ANIMALS

### ROUTE RATING

| | | |
|---|---|---|
| DIFFICULTY | | ☆☆☆☆☆ |
| ROAD CONDITION | | ☆☆☆☆☆ |
| ENVIRONMENT | | ☆☆☆☆☆ |

**ADDITIONAL NOTES**

|  | DATE |
|---|---|
|  | TIME |
|  | ROUTE |

## WEATHER CONDITIONS

| 🌡️ | ___ | ☀️ | ⛅ | 🌧️ | ⛈️ | ❄️ |
|---|---|---|---|---|---|---|
| 🎐 | ___ | ☐ | ☐ | ☐ | ☐ | ☐ |

|  | DISTANCE |
|---|---|
|  | DURATION |
|  | AVG SPEED |
|  | MAX SPEED |
|  | ELEVATION GAIN |

## BIKE SET-UP

|  | BICYCLE TYPE |
|---|---|
|  |  |
|  | EQUIPMENT & EXTRAS |
|  |  |

## ROUTE HIGHLIGHTS

| 🚩 MILESTONES & STOPS | 📍 TIME & DISTANCE | 📝 NOTES |
|---|---|---|
|  |  |  |
|  |  |  |
|  |  |  |
|  |  |  |
|  |  |  |

## ENVIRONMENT

|  | PLANTS |
|---|---|
|  |  |
|  |  |
|  | ANIMALS |
|  |  |
|  |  |

## ROUTE RATING

| 🏆 DIFFICULTY | ☆☆☆☆☆ |
|---|---|
| 🛣️ ROAD CONDITION | ☆☆☆☆☆ |
| 🏞️ ENVIRONMENT | ☆☆☆☆☆ |

### ADDITIONAL NOTES

| DATE | | WEATHER CONDITIONS | |
|---|---|---|---|
| TIME | | 🌡 ___ ☀ ⛅ 🌧 ⛈ ❄ | |
| ROUTE | | 🚩 ___ ☐ ☐ ☐ ☐ ☐ | |

| | | BIKE SET-UP | |
|---|---|---|---|
| DISTANCE | | BICYCLE TYPE | |
| DURATION | | | |
| AVG SPEED | | EQUIPMENT & EXTRAS | |
| MAX SPEED | | | |
| ELEVATION GAIN | | | |

## ROUTE HIGHLIGHTS

| MILESTONES & STOPS | TIME & DISTANCE | NOTES |
|---|---|---|
| | | |
| | | |
| | | |
| | | |
| | | |

## ENVIRONMENT

| PLANTS |
|---|
| |
| |
| ANIMALS |
| |
| |

## ROUTE RATING

| DIFFICULTY | ☆☆☆☆☆ |
|---|---|
| ROAD CONDITION | ☆☆☆☆☆ |
| ENVIRONMENT | ☆☆☆☆☆ |

### ADDITIONAL NOTES

|  | DATE |
|---|---|
|  | TIME |
|  | ROUTE |

## WEATHER CONDITIONS

| 🌡 | — | ☀ | ⛅ | 🌧 | ⛈ | ❄ |
|---|---|---|---|---|---|---|
| 🪁 | — | ☐ | ☐ | ☐ | ☐ | ☐ |

|  | DISTANCE |
|---|---|
|  | DURATION |
|  | AVG SPEED |
|  | MAX SPEED |
|  | ELEVATION GAIN |

## BIKE SET-UP

|  | BICYCLE TYPE |
|---|---|
|  |  |
|  | EQUIPMENT & EXTRAS |
|  |  |

## ROUTE HIGHLIGHTS

| MILESTONES & STOPS | TIME & DISTANCE | NOTES |
|---|---|---|
|  |  |  |
|  |  |  |
|  |  |  |
|  |  |  |
|  |  |  |

## ENVIRONMENT

| PLANTS |
|---|
|  |
|  |
| ANIMALS |
|  |
|  |

## ROUTE RATING

| DIFFICULTY | ☆☆☆☆☆ |
|---|---|
| ROAD CONDITION | ☆☆☆☆☆ |
| ENVIRONMENT | ☆☆☆☆☆ |

### ADDITIONAL NOTES

| DATE |
|---|
| TIME |
| ROUTE |

## WEATHER CONDITIONS

🌡 ____   ☀  ⛅  🌧  ⛈  ❄
🚩 ____   ☐  ☐  ☐  ☐  ☐

| DISTANCE |
|---|
| DURATION |
| AVG SPEED |
| MAX SPEED |
| ELEVATION GAIN |

## BIKE SET-UP

| BICYCLE TYPE |
|---|
| EQUIPMENT & EXTRAS |

## ROUTE HIGHLIGHTS

| MILESTONES & STOPS | TIME & DISTANCE | NOTES |
|---|---|---|
|  |  |  |
|  |  |  |
|  |  |  |
|  |  |  |
|  |  |  |

## ENVIRONMENT

| PLANTS |
|---|
|  |
|  |
| ANIMALS |
|  |
|  |

## ROUTE RATING

| DIFFICULTY | ☆☆☆☆☆ |
|---|---|
| ROAD CONDITION | ☆☆☆☆☆ |
| ENVIRONMENT | ☆☆☆☆☆ |

### ADDITIONAL NOTES

|  |  |
|---|---|
| DATE |  |
| TIME |  |
| ROUTE |  |

## WEATHER CONDITIONS

| 🌡️ ___ | ☀️ ☐ | ⛅ ☐ | 🌧️ ☐ | ⛈️ ☐ | ❄️ ☐ |
|---|---|---|---|---|---|
| 🚩 ___ | | | | | |

|  |  |
|---|---|
| DISTANCE |  |
| DURATION |  |
| AVG SPEED |  |
| MAX SPEED |  |
| ELEVATION GAIN |  |

## BIKE SET-UP

| BICYCLE TYPE |  |
|---|---|
| EQUIPMENT & EXTRAS |  |

## ROUTE HIGHLIGHTS

| MILESTONES & STOPS | TIME & DISTANCE | NOTES |
|---|---|---|
|  |  |  |
|  |  |  |
|  |  |  |
|  |  |  |
|  |  |  |

## ENVIRONMENT

| PLANTS |  |
|---|---|
| ANIMALS |  |

## ROUTE RATING

| DIFFICULTY | ☆☆☆☆☆ |
|---|---|
| ROAD CONDITION | ☆☆☆☆☆ |
| ENVIRONMENT | ☆☆☆☆☆ |

### ADDITIONAL NOTES

|  | DATE |
|---|---|
|  | TIME |
|  | ROUTE |

## WEATHER CONDITIONS

🌡 ___  ☀ ⛅ 🌧 ⛈ ❄
🪁 ___  ☐ ☐ ☐ ☐ ☐

|  | DISTANCE |
|---|---|
|  | DURATION |
|  | AVG SPEED |
|  | MAX SPEED |
|  | ELEVATION GAIN |

## BIKE SET-UP

|  | BICYCLE TYPE |
|---|---|
|  | EQUIPMENT & EXTRAS |

## ROUTE HIGHLIGHTS

| 🚩 MILESTONES & STOPS | 📍 TIME & DISTANCE | 📝 NOTES |
|---|---|---|
|  |  |  |
|  |  |  |
|  |  |  |
|  |  |  |
|  |  |  |

## ENVIRONMENT

|  | PLANTS |
|---|---|
|  |  |
|  | ANIMALS |
|  |  |

## ROUTE RATING

|  | DIFFICULTY | ☆☆☆☆☆ |
|---|---|---|
|  | ROAD CONDITION | ☆☆☆☆☆ |
|  | ENVIRONMENT | ☆☆☆☆☆ |

### ADDITIONAL NOTES

| DATE |
|---|
| TIME |
| ROUTE |

## WEATHER CONDITIONS

🌡 ____  ☀ ⛅ 🌧 ⛈ ❄
🪁 ____  ☐ ☐ ☐ ☐ ☐

| DISTANCE |
|---|
| DURATION |
| AVG SPEED |
| MAX SPEED |
| ELEVATION GAIN |

## BIKE SET-UP

| BICYCLE TYPE |
|---|
| |
| EQUIPMENT & EXTRAS |
| |

## ROUTE HIGHLIGHTS

| MILESTONES & STOPS | TIME & DISTANCE | NOTES |
|---|---|---|
| | | |
| | | |
| | | |
| | | |
| | | |

## ENVIRONMENT

| PLANTS |
|---|
| |
| |
| ANIMALS |
| |
| |

## ROUTE RATING

| | |
|---|---|
| DIFFICULTY | ☆☆☆☆☆ |
| ROAD CONDITION | ☆☆☆☆☆ |
| ENVIRONMENT | ☆☆☆☆☆ |

### ADDITIONAL NOTES

| DATE |
|---|
| TIME |
| ROUTE |

## WEATHER CONDITIONS

🌡️ ——  ☀️  ⛅  🌧️  ⛈️  ❄️
🌬️ ——  ☐  ☐  ☐  ☐  ☐

| DISTANCE |
|---|
| DURATION |
| AVG SPEED |
| MAX SPEED |
| ELEVATION GAIN |

## BIKE SET-UP

BICYCLE TYPE

EQUIPMENT & EXTRAS

## ROUTE HIGHLIGHTS

| MILESTONES & STOPS | TIME & DISTANCE | NOTES |
|---|---|---|
|  |  |  |
|  |  |  |
|  |  |  |
|  |  |  |
|  |  |  |

## ENVIRONMENT

PLANTS

ANIMALS

## ROUTE RATING

| DIFFICULTY | ☆☆☆☆☆ |
|---|---|
| ROAD CONDITION | ☆☆☆☆☆ |
| ENVIRONMENT | ☆☆☆☆☆ |

### ADDITIONAL NOTES

## DATE
## TIME
## ROUTE

## WEATHER CONDITIONS

## DISTANCE
## DURATION
## AVG SPEED
## MAX SPEED
## ELEVATION GAIN

## BIKE SET-UP

BICYCLE TYPE

EQUIPMENT & EXTRAS

## ROUTE HIGHLIGHTS

| MILESTONES & STOPS | TIME & DISTANCE | NOTES |
|---|---|---|
|  |  |  |
|  |  |  |
|  |  |  |
|  |  |  |
|  |  |  |

## ENVIRONMENT

PLANTS

ANIMALS

## ROUTE RATING

DIFFICULTY ☆☆☆☆☆

ROAD CONDITION ☆☆☆☆☆

ENVIRONMENT ☆☆☆☆☆

### ADDITIONAL NOTES

|  |  |
|---|---|
| 📅 DATE |  |
| 🕐 TIME |  |
| 🗺️ ROUTE |  |

## WEATHER CONDITIONS

| 🌡️ | ___ | ☀️ | ⛅ | 🌧️ | ⛈️ | ❄️ |
|---|---|---|---|---|---|---|
| 🚩 | ___ | ☐ | ☐ | ☐ | ☐ | ☐ |

|  |  |
|---|---|
| 📍 DISTANCE |  |
| ⏱️ DURATION |  |
| 🎯 AVG SPEED |  |
| 🚴 MAX SPEED |  |
| ⛰️ ELEVATION GAIN |  |

## BIKE SET-UP

| 🚲 BICYCLE TYPE |  |
|---|---|
| 🎒 EQUIPMENT & EXTRAS |  |

## ROUTE HIGHLIGHTS

| 🚩 MILESTONES & STOPS | 📍 TIME & DISTANCE | 📝 NOTES |
|---|---|---|
|  |  |  |
|  |  |  |
|  |  |  |
|  |  |  |
|  |  |  |

## ENVIRONMENT

| 🌿 PLANTS |  |
|---|---|
|  |  |
|  |  |
| 🦆 ANIMALS |  |
|  |  |
|  |  |

## ROUTE RATING

| 🏆 DIFFICULTY | ☆☆☆☆☆ |
|---|---|
| 🛣️ ROAD CONDITION | ☆☆☆☆☆ |
| 🌄 ENVIRONMENT | ☆☆☆☆☆ |

### ADDITIONAL NOTES

| DATE |
|---|
| TIME |
| ROUTE |

## WEATHER CONDITIONS

🌡️ _____  ☀️ ⛅ 🌧️ ⛈️ ❄️
🚩 _____  ☐ ☐ ☐ ☐ ☐

| DISTANCE |
|---|
| DURATION |
| AVG SPEED |
| MAX SPEED |
| ELEVATION GAIN |

## BIKE SET-UP

BICYCLE TYPE

EQUIPMENT & EXTRAS

## ROUTE HIGHLIGHTS

| MILESTONES & STOPS | TIME & DISTANCE | NOTES |
|---|---|---|
|  |  |  |
|  |  |  |
|  |  |  |
|  |  |  |
|  |  |  |

## ENVIRONMENT

PLANTS



ANIMALS

## ROUTE RATING

| DIFFICULTY | ☆☆☆☆☆ |
|---|---|
| ROAD CONDITION | ☆☆☆☆☆ |
| ENVIRONMENT | ☆☆☆☆☆ |

### ADDITIONAL NOTES

## Ride Log

|  |  |
|---|---|
| 📅 DATE | |
| 🕐 TIME | |
| 🗺️ ROUTE | |

### WEATHER CONDITIONS

🌡️ _____  ☀️  ⛅  🌧️  ⛈️  ❄️
🚩 _____  ☐  ☐  ☐  ☐  ☐

|  |  |
|---|---|
| 📍 DISTANCE | |
| ⏱️ DURATION | |
| 🏁 AVG SPEED | |
| 🚜 MAX SPEED | |
| ⛰️ ELEVATION GAIN | |

### BIKE SET-UP

| 🚲 BICYCLE TYPE | |
|---|---|
| 🎒 EQUIPMENT & EXTRAS | |

### ROUTE HIGHLIGHTS

| 🚩 MILESTONES & STOPS | 📍 TIME & DISTANCE | 📝 NOTES |
|---|---|---|
|  |  |  |
|  |  |  |
|  |  |  |
|  |  |  |
|  |  |  |

### ENVIRONMENT

| 🌳 PLANTS | |
|---|---|
|  | |
| 🦆 ANIMALS | |
|  | |

### ROUTE RATING

| 🏆 DIFFICULTY | ☆☆☆☆☆ |
|---|---|
| 🛣️ ROAD CONDITION | ☆☆☆☆☆ |
| ⛰️ ENVIRONMENT | ☆☆☆☆☆ |

### ADDITIONAL NOTES

|  | DATE |
|---|---|
|  | TIME |
|  | ROUTE |

## WEATHER CONDITIONS

| 🌡️ | ― | ☀️ | ⛅ | 🌧️ | ⛈️ | ❄️ |
|---|---|---|---|---|---|---|
| 🚩 | ― | ☐ | ☐ | ☐ | ☐ | ☐ |

|  | DISTANCE |
|---|---|
|  | DURATION |
|  | AVG SPEED |
|  | MAX SPEED |
|  | ELEVATION GAIN |

## BIKE SET-UP

|  | BICYCLE TYPE |
|---|---|
|  |  |
|  | EQUIPMENT & EXTRAS |
|  |  |

## ROUTE HIGHLIGHTS

| MILESTONES & STOPS | TIME & DISTANCE | NOTES |
|---|---|---|
|  |  |  |
|  |  |  |
|  |  |  |
|  |  |  |
|  |  |  |

## ENVIRONMENT

| PLANTS |
|---|
|  |
|  |
| ANIMALS |
|  |
|  |

## ROUTE RATING

| DIFFICULTY | ☆☆☆☆☆ |
|---|---|
| ROAD CONDITION | ☆☆☆☆☆ |
| ENVIRONMENT | ☆☆☆☆☆ |

### ADDITIONAL NOTES

| | |
|---|---|
| 📅 DATE | |
| 🕐 TIME | |
| 🗺️ ROUTE | |

## WEATHER CONDITIONS

| 🌡️ | ___ | ☀️ | ⛅ | 🌧️ | ⛈️ | ❄️ |
|---|---|---|---|---|---|---|
| 🚩 | ___ | ☐ | ☐ | ☐ | ☐ | ☐ |

| | |
|---|---|
| 📍 DISTANCE | |
| ⏱️ DURATION | |
| 🌡️ AVG SPEED | |
| 🚴 MAX SPEED | |
| ⛰️ ELEVATION GAIN | |

## BIKE SET-UP

| | |
|---|---|
| 🚲 BICYCLE TYPE | |
| 🧤 EQUIPMENT & EXTRAS | |

## ROUTE HIGHLIGHTS

| 🚩 MILESTONES & STOPS | 📍 TIME & DISTANCE | 📋 NOTES |
|---|---|---|
| | | |
| | | |
| | | |
| | | |
| | | |

## ENVIRONMENT

| | |
|---|---|
| 🌳 PLANTS | |
| 🦆 ANIMALS | |

## ROUTE RATING

| | | |
|---|---|---|
| 🏆 DIFFICULTY | | ☆☆☆☆☆ |
| 🛣️ ROAD CONDITION | | ☆☆☆☆☆ |
| 🏞️ ENVIRONMENT | | ☆☆☆☆☆ |

### ADDITIONAL NOTES

| DATE |
|---|
| TIME |
| ROUTE |

## WEATHER CONDITIONS

🌡️ _____  ☀️  ⛅  🌧️  ⛈️  ❄️

🚩 _____  ☐  ☐  ☐  ☐

| DISTANCE |
|---|
| DURATION |
| AVG SPEED |
| MAX SPEED |
| ELEVATION GAIN |

## BIKE SET-UP

| BICYCLE TYPE |
|---|
| |
| EQUIPMENT & EXTRAS |
| |

## ROUTE HIGHLIGHTS

| MILESTONES & STOPS | TIME & DISTANCE | NOTES |
|---|---|---|
| | | |
| | | |
| | | |
| | | |
| | | |

## ENVIRONMENT

| PLANTS |
|---|
| |
| |
| ANIMALS |
| |
| |

## ROUTE RATING

| DIFFICULTY | ☆☆☆☆☆ |
|---|---|
| ROAD CONDITION | ☆☆☆☆☆ |
| ENVIRONMENT | ☆☆☆☆☆ |

### ADDITIONAL NOTES

| DATE | | | WEATHER CONDITIONS | |
|---|---|---|---|---|
| TIME | | | 🌡 ___ ☀ ⛅ 🌧 ⛈ ❄ | |
| ROUTE | | | 🚩 ___ ☐ ☐ ☐ ☐ ☐ | |

| DISTANCE |
|---|
| DURATION |
| AVG SPEED |
| MAX SPEED |
| ELEVATION GAIN |

| BIKE SET-UP |
|---|
| BICYCLE TYPE |
| |
| EQUIPMENT & EXTRAS |
| |

## ROUTE HIGHLIGHTS

| MILESTONES & STOPS | TIME & DISTANCE | NOTES |
|---|---|---|
| | | |
| | | |
| | | |
| | | |
| | | |

## ENVIRONMENT

| PLANTS |
|---|
| |
| |
| ANIMALS |
| |
| |

## ROUTE RATING

| DIFFICULTY | ☆☆☆☆☆ |
|---|---|
| ROAD CONDITION | ☆☆☆☆☆ |
| ENVIRONMENT | ☆☆☆☆☆ |

### ADDITIONAL NOTES

| DATE | |
|---|---|
| TIME | |
| ROUTE | |

## WEATHER CONDITIONS

🌡️ _____  ☀️  ⛅  🌧️  ⛈️  ❄️
🚩 _____  ☐   ☐   ☐   ☐   ☐

| DISTANCE | |
|---|---|
| DURATION | |
| AVG SPEED | |
| MAX SPEED | |
| ELEVATION GAIN | |

## BIKE SET-UP

| BICYCLE TYPE | |
|---|---|
| | |
| EQUIPMENT & EXTRAS | |
| | |

## ROUTE HIGHLIGHTS

| MILESTONES & STOPS | TIME & DISTANCE | NOTES |
|---|---|---|
| | | |
| | | |
| | | |
| | | |
| | | |

## ENVIRONMENT

| PLANTS | |
|---|---|
| | |
| | |
| ANIMALS | |
| | |
| | |

## ROUTE RATING

| DIFFICULTY | ☆☆☆☆☆ |
|---|---|
| ROAD CONDITION | ☆☆☆☆☆ |
| ENVIRONMENT | ☆☆☆☆☆ |

### ADDITIONAL NOTES

|  |  |
|---|---|
| 📅 DATE |  |
| 🕐 TIME |  |
| 🗺️ ROUTE |  |

## WEATHER CONDITIONS

| 🌡️ | ___ | ☀️ | ⛅ | 🌧️ | ⛈️ | ❄️ |
|---|---|---|---|---|---|---|
| 🪁 | ___ | ☐ | ☐ | ☐ | ☐ | ☐ |

|  |  |
|---|---|
| 📍 DISTANCE |  |
| ⏱️ DURATION |  |
| 🎚️ AVG SPEED |  |
| 🚴 MAX SPEED |  |
| ⛰️ ELEVATION GAIN |  |

## BIKE SET-UP

|  |  |
|---|---|
| 🚲 BICYCLE TYPE |  |
| 🧤 EQUIPMENT & EXTRAS |  |

## ROUTE HIGHLIGHTS

| 🚩 MILESTONES & STOPS | 📍 TIME & DISTANCE | 📝 NOTES |
|---|---|---|
|  |  |  |
|  |  |  |
|  |  |  |
|  |  |  |
|  |  |  |

## ENVIRONMENT

| 🌿 PLANTS |
|---|
|  |
|  |
| 🦆 ANIMALS |
|  |
|  |

## ROUTE RATING

|  |  |  |
|---|---|---|
| 🏆 DIFFICULTY | ☆☆☆☆☆ |
| 🛣️ ROAD CONDITION | ☆☆☆☆☆ |
| 🏞️ ENVIRONMENT | ☆☆☆☆☆ |

### ADDITIONAL NOTES

## DATE
## TIME
## ROUTE

## WEATHER CONDITIONS

## DISTANCE
## DURATION
## AVG SPEED
## MAX SPEED
## ELEVATION GAIN

## BIKE SET-UP
BICYCLE TYPE

EQUIPMENT & EXTRAS

## ROUTE HIGHLIGHTS

| MILESTONES & STOPS | TIME & DISTANCE | NOTES |
|---|---|---|
|  |  |  |
|  |  |  |
|  |  |  |
|  |  |  |
|  |  |  |

## ENVIRONMENT

PLANTS

ANIMALS

## ROUTE RATING

DIFFICULTY ☆☆☆☆☆

ROAD CONDITION ☆☆☆☆☆

ENVIRONMENT ☆☆☆☆☆

### ADDITIONAL NOTES

| | DATE |
|---|---|
| | TIME |
| | ROUTE |

## WEATHER CONDITIONS

| 🌡 | ___ | ☀ | ⛅ | 🌧 | ⛈ | ❄ |
|---|---|---|---|---|---|---|
| 🚩 | ___ | ☐ | ☐ | ☐ | ☐ | ☐ |

| | DISTANCE |
|---|---|
| | DURATION |
| | AVG SPEED |
| | MAX SPEED |
| | ELEVATION GAIN |

## BIKE SET-UP

| | BICYCLE TYPE |
|---|---|
| | |
| | EQUIPMENT & EXTRAS |
| | |

## ROUTE HIGHLIGHTS

| MILESTONES & STOPS | TIME & DISTANCE | NOTES |
|---|---|---|
| | | |
| | | |
| | | |
| | | |
| | | |

## ENVIRONMENT

| | PLANTS |
|---|---|
| | |
| | ANIMALS |
| | |

## ROUTE RATING

| | DIFFICULTY | ☆☆☆☆☆ |
|---|---|---|
| | ROAD CONDITION | ☆☆☆☆☆ |
| | ENVIRONMENT | ☆☆☆☆☆ |

### ADDITIONAL NOTES

| DATE |
|---|
| TIME |
| ROUTE |

## WEATHER CONDITIONS

🌡 ____  ☀️  ⛅  🌧  ⛈  ❄️

🚩 ____  ☐  ☐  ☐  ☐  ☐

| DISTANCE |
|---|
| DURATION |
| AVG SPEED |
| MAX SPEED |
| ELEVATION GAIN |

## BIKE SET-UP

| BICYCLE TYPE |
|---|
|  |
| EQUIPMENT & EXTRAS |
|  |

## ROUTE HIGHLIGHTS

| MILESTONES & STOPS | TIME & DISTANCE | NOTES |
|---|---|---|
|  |  |  |
|  |  |  |
|  |  |  |
|  |  |  |
|  |  |  |

## ENVIRONMENT

| PLANTS |
|---|
|  |
| ANIMALS |
|  |

## ROUTE RATING

| DIFFICULTY | ☆☆☆☆☆ |
|---|---|
| ROAD CONDITION | ☆☆☆☆☆ |
| ENVIRONMENT | ☆☆☆☆☆ |

### ADDITIONAL NOTES

| DATE |
|---|
| TIME |
| ROUTE |

| WEATHER CONDITIONS |
|---|
| 🌡 ___  ☀ ⛅ 🌧 ⛈ ❄ |
| 🚩 ___  ☐ ☐ ☐ ☐ ☐ |

| DISTANCE |
|---|
| DURATION |
| AVG SPEED |
| MAX SPEED |
| ELEVATION GAIN |

| BIKE SET-UP |
|---|
| BICYCLE TYPE |
| EQUIPMENT & EXTRAS |

## ROUTE HIGHLIGHTS

| MILESTONES & STOPS | TIME & DISTANCE | NOTES |
|---|---|---|
|  |  |  |
|  |  |  |
|  |  |  |
|  |  |  |
|  |  |  |

## ENVIRONMENT

| PLANTS |
|---|
|  |
|  |
| ANIMALS |
|  |
|  |

## ROUTE RATING

| DIFFICULTY | ☆☆☆☆☆ |
|---|---|
| ROAD CONDITION | ☆☆☆☆☆ |
| ENVIRONMENT | ☆☆☆☆☆ |

### ADDITIONAL NOTES

| DATE |
|---|
| TIME |
| ROUTE |

## WEATHER CONDITIONS

🌡 ___  ☀ ⛅ 🌧 ⛈ ❄
🚩 ___  ☐ ☐ ☐ ☐ ☐

| |
|---|
| DISTANCE |
| DURATION |
| AVG SPEED |
| MAX SPEED |
| ELEVATION GAIN |

## BIKE SET-UP

| |
|---|
| BICYCLE TYPE |
| |
| EQUIPMENT & EXTRAS |
| |

## ROUTE HIGHLIGHTS

| MILESTONES & STOPS | TIME & DISTANCE | NOTES |
|---|---|---|
| | | |
| | | |
| | | |
| | | |
| | | |

## ENVIRONMENT

| |
|---|
| PLANTS |
| |
| |
| ANIMALS |
| |
| |

## ROUTE RATING

| | |
|---|---|
| DIFFICULTY | ☆☆☆☆☆ |
| ROAD CONDITION | ☆☆☆☆☆ |
| ENVIRONMENT | ☆☆☆☆☆ |

### ADDITIONAL NOTES

|  | DATE |
|---|---|
|  | TIME |
|  | ROUTE |

## WEATHER CONDITIONS

| 🌡 | ___ | ☀ | ⛅ | 🌧 | ⛈ | ❄ |
|---|---|---|---|---|---|---|
| 🚩 | ___ | ☐ | ☐ | ☐ | ☐ | ☐ |

|  | DISTANCE |
|---|---|
|  | DURATION |
|  | AVG SPEED |
|  | MAX SPEED |
|  | ELEVATION GAIN |

## BIKE SET-UP

|  | BICYCLE TYPE |
|---|---|
|  | EQUIPMENT & EXTRAS |

## ROUTE HIGHLIGHTS

| MILESTONES & STOPS | TIME & DISTANCE | NOTES |
|---|---|---|
|  |  |  |
|  |  |  |
|  |  |  |
|  |  |  |
|  |  |  |

## ENVIRONMENT

| PLANTS |
|---|
|  |
| ANIMALS |
|  |

## ROUTE RATING

| DIFFICULTY | ☆☆☆☆☆ |
|---|---|
| ROAD CONDITION | ☆☆☆☆☆ |
| ENVIRONMENT | ☆☆☆☆☆ |

### ADDITIONAL NOTES

| DATE |
|---|
| TIME |
| ROUTE |

| WEATHER CONDITIONS |
|---|
| 🌡 ____  ☀ ⛅ 🌧 ⛈ ❄ |
| 🚩 ____  ☐ ☐ ☐ ☐ ☐ |

| DISTANCE |
|---|
| DURATION |
| AVG SPEED |
| MAX SPEED |
| ELEVATION GAIN |

| BIKE SET-UP |
|---|
| BICYCLE TYPE |
| |
| EQUIPMENT & EXTRAS |
| |

### ROUTE HIGHLIGHTS

| MILESTONES & STOPS | TIME & DISTANCE | NOTES |
|---|---|---|
| | | |
| | | |
| | | |
| | | |
| | | |

### ENVIRONMENT

| PLANTS |
|---|
| |
| |
| ANIMALS |
| |
| |

### ROUTE RATING

| DIFFICULTY | ☆☆☆☆☆ |
|---|---|
| ROAD CONDITION | ☆☆☆☆☆ |
| ENVIRONMENT | ☆☆☆☆☆ |

| ADDITIONAL NOTES |
|---|
| |
| |

| DATE |
|---|
| TIME |
| ROUTE |

| WEATHER CONDITIONS |
|---|
| 🌡️ ____  ☀️ ⛅ 🌧️ ⛈️ ❄️ |
| 🌬️ ____  ☐ ☐ ☐ ☐ ☐ |

| DISTANCE |
|---|
| DURATION |
| AVG SPEED |
| MAX SPEED |
| ELEVATION GAIN |

| BIKE SET-UP |
|---|
| BICYCLE TYPE |
| |
| EQUIPMENT & EXTRAS |
| |

## ROUTE HIGHLIGHTS

| MILESTONES & STOPS | TIME & DISTANCE | NOTES |
|---|---|---|
|  |  |  |
|  |  |  |
|  |  |  |
|  |  |  |
|  |  |  |

## ENVIRONMENT

| PLANTS |
|---|
|  |
|  |
| ANIMALS |
|  |
|  |

## ROUTE RATING

| DIFFICULTY | ☆☆☆☆☆ |
|---|---|
| ROAD CONDITION | ☆☆☆☆☆ |
| ENVIRONMENT | ☆☆☆☆☆ |

### ADDITIONAL NOTES

| DATE |
|---|
| TIME |
| ROUTE |

## WEATHER CONDITIONS

🌡️ ——  ☀️  ⛅  🌧️  ⛈️  ❄️
🍃 ——  ☐  ☐  ☐  ☐  ☐

| DISTANCE |
|---|
| DURATION |
| AVG SPEED |
| MAX SPEED |
| ELEVATION GAIN |

## BIKE SET-UP

| BICYCLE TYPE |
|---|
| EQUIPMENT & EXTRAS |

## ROUTE HIGHLIGHTS

| MILESTONES & STOPS | TIME & DISTANCE | NOTES |
|---|---|---|
|  |  |  |
|  |  |  |
|  |  |  |
|  |  |  |
|  |  |  |

## ENVIRONMENT

| PLANTS |
|---|
|  |
|  |
| ANIMALS |
|  |
|  |

## ROUTE RATING

| DIFFICULTY | ☆☆☆☆☆ |
|---|---|
| ROAD CONDITION | ☆☆☆☆☆ |
| ENVIRONMENT | ☆☆☆☆☆ |

### ADDITIONAL NOTES

| DATE |
|---|
| TIME |
| ROUTE |

## WEATHER CONDITIONS

🌡 ____  ☀ ☁ 🌧 ⛈ ❄
🚩 ____  ☐ ☐ ☐ ☐ ☐

| DISTANCE |
|---|
| DURATION |
| AVG SPEED |
| MAX SPEED |
| ELEVATION GAIN |

## BIKE SET-UP

| BICYCLE TYPE |
|---|
| |
| EQUIPMENT & EXTRAS |
| |

## ROUTE HIGHLIGHTS

| MILESTONES & STOPS | TIME & DISTANCE | NOTES |
|---|---|---|
| | | |
| | | |
| | | |
| | | |
| | | |

## ENVIRONMENT

| PLANTS |
|---|
| |
| |
| ANIMALS |
| |
| |

## ROUTE RATING

| DIFFICULTY | ☆☆☆☆☆ |
|---|---|
| ROAD CONDITION | ☆☆☆☆☆ |
| ENVIRONMENT | ☆☆☆☆☆ |

### ADDITIONAL NOTES

| |
|---|
| |

|  | DATE |
|---|---|
|  | TIME |
|  | ROUTE |

|  | DISTANCE |
|---|---|
|  | DURATION |
|  | AVG SPEED |
|  | MAX SPEED |
|  | ELEVATION GAIN |

## WEATHER CONDITIONS

🌡 _____  ☀  ⛅  🌧  ⛈  ❄
🚩 _____  ☐  ☐  ☐  ☐  ☐

## BIKE SET-UP

|  | BICYCLE TYPE |
|---|---|
|  | EQUIPMENT & EXTRAS |

## ROUTE HIGHLIGHTS

| MILESTONES & STOPS | TIME & DISTANCE | NOTES |
|---|---|---|
|  |  |  |
|  |  |  |
|  |  |  |
|  |  |  |
|  |  |  |

## ENVIRONMENT

|  | PLANTS |
|---|---|
|  |  |
|  | ANIMALS |
|  |  |

## ROUTE RATING

| | | |
|---|---|---|
| 🏆 | DIFFICULTY | ☆☆☆☆☆ |
| 🛣 | ROAD CONDITION | ☆☆☆☆☆ |
| 🏞 | ENVIRONMENT | ☆☆☆☆☆ |

### ADDITIONAL NOTES

|  | DATE |
|---|---|
|  | TIME |
|  | ROUTE |

| WEATHER CONDITIONS | | | | | |
|---|---|---|---|---|---|
| 🌡 ___ | ☀ | ⛅ | 🌧 | ⛈ | ❄ |
| 🚩 ___ | ☐ | ☐ | ☐ | ☐ | ☐ |

|  | DISTANCE |
|---|---|
|  | DURATION |
|  | AVG SPEED |
|  | MAX SPEED |
|  | ELEVATION GAIN |

| BIKE SET-UP |
|---|
| BICYCLE TYPE |
|  |
| EQUIPMENT & EXTRAS |
|  |

## ROUTE HIGHLIGHTS

| 🚩 MILESTONES & STOPS | 📍 TIME & DISTANCE | 📝 NOTES |
|---|---|---|
|  |  |  |
|  |  |  |
|  |  |  |
|  |  |  |
|  |  |  |

### ENVIRONMENT

| PLANTS |
|---|
|  |
|  |
| ANIMALS |
|  |
|  |

### ROUTE RATING

| DIFFICULTY | ☆☆☆☆☆ |
|---|---|
| ROAD CONDITION | ☆☆☆☆☆ |
| ENVIRONMENT | ☆☆☆☆☆ |

| ADDITIONAL NOTES |
|---|
|  |
|  |

| DATE | |
|---|---|
| TIME | |
| ROUTE | |

## WEATHER CONDITIONS

🌡️ _____  ☀️  ⛅  🌧️  ⛈️  ❄️
🪁 _____  ☐   ☐   ☐   ☐   ☐

| DISTANCE | |
|---|---|
| DURATION | |
| AVG SPEED | |
| MAX SPEED | |
| ELEVATION GAIN | |

## BIKE SET-UP

| BICYCLE TYPE | |
|---|---|
| | |
| EQUIPMENT & EXTRAS | |
| | |

## ROUTE HIGHLIGHTS

| MILESTONES & STOPS | TIME & DISTANCE | NOTES |
|---|---|---|
| | | |
| | | |
| | | |
| | | |
| | | |

## ENVIRONMENT

| PLANTS | |
|---|---|
| | |
| | |
| ANIMALS | |
| | |
| | |

## ROUTE RATING

| DIFFICULTY | ☆☆☆☆☆ |
|---|---|
| ROAD CONDITION | ☆☆☆☆☆ |
| ENVIRONMENT | ☆☆☆☆☆ |

### ADDITIONAL NOTES

|  |  |
|---|---|
| 📅 DATE | |
| 🕐 TIME | |
| 🗺️ ROUTE | |

## WEATHER CONDITIONS

| 🌡️ ____ | ☀️ | ⛅ | 🌧️ | ⛈️ | ❄️ |
|---|---|---|---|---|---|
| 🪁 ____ | ☐ | ☐ | ☐ | ☐ | ☐ |

|  |
|---|
| 📍 DISTANCE |
| ⏱️ DURATION |
| 🚴 AVG SPEED |
| 🚲 MAX SPEED |
| ⛰️ ELEVATION GAIN |

## BIKE SET-UP

| 🚲 BICYCLE TYPE |
|---|
|  |
| 🎒 EQUIPMENT & EXTRAS |
|  |

## ROUTE HIGHLIGHTS

| 🚩 MILESTONES & STOPS | 📍 TIME & DISTANCE | 📝 NOTES |
|---|---|---|
|  |  |  |
|  |  |  |
|  |  |  |
|  |  |  |
|  |  |  |

## ENVIRONMENT

| 🌿 PLANTS |
|---|
|  |
|  |
| 🦆 ANIMALS |
|  |
|  |

## ROUTE RATING

| 🏆 DIFFICULTY | ☆☆☆☆☆ |
|---|---|
| 🛣️ ROAD CONDITION | ☆☆☆☆☆ |
| 🏞️ ENVIRONMENT | ☆☆☆☆☆ |

### ADDITIONAL NOTES

| DATE | |
|---|---|
| TIME | |
| ROUTE | |

## WEATHER CONDITIONS

Temperature: ___
Wind: ___

☀ ⛅ 🌧 ⛈ ❄
☐ ☐ ☐ ☐ ☐

| DISTANCE | |
|---|---|
| DURATION | |
| AVG SPEED | |
| MAX SPEED | |
| ELEVATION GAIN | |

## BIKE SET-UP

| BICYCLE TYPE | |
|---|---|
| EQUIPMENT & EXTRAS | |

## ROUTE HIGHLIGHTS

| MILESTONES & STOPS | TIME & DISTANCE | NOTES |
|---|---|---|
| | | |
| | | |
| | | |
| | | |
| | | |

## ENVIRONMENT

| PLANTS | |
|---|---|
| ANIMALS | |

## ROUTE RATING

| DIFFICULTY | ☆☆☆☆☆ |
|---|---|
| ROAD CONDITION | ☆☆☆☆☆ |
| ENVIRONMENT | ☆☆☆☆☆ |

### ADDITIONAL NOTES

| DATE |
|---|
| TIME |
| ROUTE |

## WEATHER CONDITIONS

🌡️ _____ ☀️ ⛅ 🌧️ ⛈️ ❄️
🚩 _____ ☐ ☐ ☐ ☐ ☐

| DISTANCE |
|---|
| DURATION |
| AVG SPEED |
| MAX SPEED |
| ELEVATION GAIN |

## BIKE SET-UP

| BICYCLE TYPE |
|---|
| |
| EQUIPMENT & EXTRAS |
| |

## ROUTE HIGHLIGHTS

| MILESTONES & STOPS | TIME & DISTANCE | NOTES |
|---|---|---|
| | | |
| | | |
| | | |
| | | |
| | | |

## ENVIRONMENT

| PLANTS |
|---|
| |
| |
| ANIMALS |
| |
| |

## ROUTE RATING

| DIFFICULTY | ☆☆☆☆☆ |
|---|---|
| ROAD CONDITION | ☆☆☆☆☆ |
| ENVIRONMENT | ☆☆☆☆☆ |

### ADDITIONAL NOTES

|  | DATE |
|---|---|
|  | TIME |
|  | ROUTE |

## WEATHER CONDITIONS

🌡️ _____  ☀️ ⛅ 🌧️ ⛈️ ❄️

🌬️ _____  ☐ ☐ ☐ ☐ ☐

|  | DISTANCE |
|---|---|
|  | DURATION |
|  | AVG SPEED |
|  | MAX SPEED |
|  | ELEVATION GAIN |

## BIKE SET-UP

| | BICYCLE TYPE |
|---|---|
| | |
| | EQUIPMENT & EXTRAS |
| | |

## ROUTE HIGHLIGHTS

| MILESTONES & STOPS | TIME & DISTANCE | NOTES |
|---|---|---|
| | | |
| | | |
| | | |
| | | |
| | | |

## ENVIRONMENT

| PLANTS |
|---|
| |
| |
| ANIMALS |
| |
| |

## ROUTE RATING

| DIFFICULTY | ☆☆☆☆☆ |
|---|---|
| ROAD CONDITION | ☆☆☆☆☆ |
| ENVIRONMENT | ☆☆☆☆☆ |

### ADDITIONAL NOTES

| DATE |
|---|
| TIME |
| ROUTE |

| WEATHER CONDITIONS |
|---|
| 🌡 ____   ☀ ⛅ 🌧 ⛈ ❄ |
| 🚩 ____   ☐ ☐ ☐ ☐ ☐ |

| DISTANCE |
|---|
| DURATION |
| AVG SPEED |
| MAX SPEED |
| ELEVATION GAIN |

| BIKE SET-UP |
|---|
| BICYCLE TYPE |
| |
| EQUIPMENT & EXTRAS |
| |

## ROUTE HIGHLIGHTS

| MILESTONES & STOPS | TIME & DISTANCE | NOTES |
|---|---|---|
| | | |
| | | |
| | | |
| | | |
| | | |

## ENVIRONMENT

| PLANTS |
|---|
| |
| |
| ANIMALS |
| |
| |

## ROUTE RATING

| DIFFICULTY | ☆☆☆☆☆ |
|---|---|
| ROAD CONDITION | ☆☆☆☆☆ |
| ENVIRONMENT | ☆☆☆☆☆ |

### ADDITIONAL NOTES

|  |  |
|---|---|
| 📅 DATE | |
| 🕐 TIME | |
| 🗺️ ROUTE | |

## WEATHER CONDITIONS

| 🌡️ ___ | ☀️ | ⛅ | 🌧️ | ⛈️ | ❄️ |
|---|---|---|---|---|---|
| 🚩 ___ | ☐ | ☐ | ☐ | ☐ | ☐ |

|  |  |
|---|---|
| 📍 DISTANCE | |
| ⏱️ DURATION | |
| 🏁 AVG SPEED | |
| 🚴 MAX SPEED | |
| ⛰️ ELEVATION GAIN | |

## BIKE SET-UP

| 🚲 BICYCLE TYPE | |
|---|---|
| 🎒 EQUIPMENT & EXTRAS | |

## ROUTE HIGHLIGHTS

| 🚩 MILESTONES & STOPS | 📍 TIME & DISTANCE | 📋 NOTES |
|---|---|---|
| | | |
| | | |
| | | |
| | | |
| | | |

## ENVIRONMENT

| 🌳 PLANTS | |
|---|---|
| | |
| | |
| 🦆 ANIMALS | |
| | |
| | |

## ROUTE RATING

| 🏆 DIFFICULTY | ☆☆☆☆☆ |
|---|---|
| 🛣️ ROAD CONDITION | ☆☆☆☆☆ |
| 🏞️ ENVIRONMENT | ☆☆☆☆☆ |

### ADDITIONAL NOTES

| |
|---|
| |

| | DATE | |
|---|---|---|
| | TIME | |
| | ROUTE | |

| WEATHER CONDITIONS | | | | | |
|---|---|---|---|---|---|
| 🌡 ___ | ☀ | ⛅ | 🌧 | ⛈ | ❄ |
| 🚩 ___ | ☐ | ☐ | ☐ | ☐ | ☐ |

| | DISTANCE | |
|---|---|---|
| | DURATION | |
| | AVG SPEED | |
| | MAX SPEED | |
| | ELEVATION GAIN | |

| BIKE SET-UP | |
|---|---|
| BICYCLE TYPE | |
| | |
| EQUIPMENT & EXTRAS | |
| | |

## ROUTE HIGHLIGHTS

| MILESTONES & STOPS | TIME & DISTANCE | NOTES |
|---|---|---|
| | | |
| | | |
| | | |
| | | |
| | | |

## ENVIRONMENT

| PLANTS | |
|---|---|
| | |
| | |
| ANIMALS | |
| | |
| | |

## ROUTE RATING

| DIFFICULTY | ☆☆☆☆☆ |
|---|---|
| ROAD CONDITION | ☆☆☆☆☆ |
| ENVIRONMENT | ☆☆☆☆☆ |

| ADDITIONAL NOTES |
|---|
| |
| |

| DATE |
|---|
| TIME |
| ROUTE |

## WEATHER CONDITIONS

🌡 ——  ☀ ⛅ 🌧 ⛈ ❄
🪁 ——  ☐ ☐ ☐ ☐ ☐

| DISTANCE |
|---|
| DURATION |
| AVG SPEED |
| MAX SPEED |
| ELEVATION GAIN |

## BIKE SET-UP

| BICYCLE TYPE |
|---|
|  |
| EQUIPMENT & EXTRAS |
|  |

## ROUTE HIGHLIGHTS

| MILESTONES & STOPS | TIME & DISTANCE | NOTES |
|---|---|---|
|  |  |  |
|  |  |  |
|  |  |  |
|  |  |  |
|  |  |  |

## ENVIRONMENT

| PLANTS |
|---|
|  |
|  |
| ANIMALS |
|  |
|  |

## ROUTE RATING

| DIFFICULTY | ☆☆☆☆☆ |
|---|---|
| ROAD CONDITION | ☆☆☆☆☆ |
| ENVIRONMENT | ☆☆☆☆☆ |

### ADDITIONAL NOTES

| DATE |
|---|
| TIME |
| ROUTE |

| WEATHER CONDITIONS |
|---|
| 🌡 ____  ☀ ⛅ 🌧 ⛈ ❄ |
| 🚩 ____  ☐ ☐ ☐ ☐ ☐ |

| DISTANCE |
|---|
| DURATION |
| AVG SPEED |
| MAX SPEED |
| ELEVATION GAIN |

| BIKE SET-UP |
|---|
| BICYCLE TYPE |
| |
| EQUIPMENT & EXTRAS |
| |

## ROUTE HIGHLIGHTS

| MILESTONES & STOPS | TIME & DISTANCE | NOTES |
|---|---|---|
|  |  |  |
|  |  |  |
|  |  |  |
|  |  |  |
|  |  |  |

## ENVIRONMENT

| PLANTS |
|---|
|  |
|  |
| ANIMALS |
|  |
|  |

## ROUTE RATING

| DIFFICULTY | ☆☆☆☆☆ |
|---|---|
| ROAD CONDITION | ☆☆☆☆☆ |
| ENVIRONMENT | ☆☆☆☆☆ |

### ADDITIONAL NOTES

## DATE

## TIME

## ROUTE

## WEATHER CONDITIONS

## DISTANCE
## DURATION
## AVG SPEED
## MAX SPEED
## ELEVATION GAIN

## BIKE SET-UP

BICYCLE TYPE

EQUIPMENT & EXTRAS

## ROUTE HIGHLIGHTS

| MILESTONES & STOPS | TIME & DISTANCE | NOTES |
|---|---|---|
|  |  |  |
|  |  |  |
|  |  |  |
|  |  |  |
|  |  |  |

## ENVIRONMENT

PLANTS

ANIMALS

## ROUTE RATING

DIFFICULTY ☆☆☆☆☆

ROAD CONDITION ☆☆☆☆☆

ENVIRONMENT ☆☆☆☆☆

### ADDITIONAL NOTES

|  | DATE |
|---|---|
|  | TIME |
|  | ROUTE |

## WEATHER CONDITIONS

|  | ☀️ | ⛅ | 🌧️ | ⛈️ | ❄️ |
|---|---|---|---|---|---|
| 🌡️ — | | | | | |
| 🚩 — | ☐ | ☐ | ☐ | ☐ | ☐ |

|  | DISTANCE |
|---|---|
|  | DURATION |
|  | AVG SPEED |
|  | MAX SPEED |
|  | ELEVATION GAIN |

## BIKE SET-UP

|  | BICYCLE TYPE |
|---|---|
|  | EQUIPMENT & EXTRAS |

## ROUTE HIGHLIGHTS

| MILESTONES & STOPS | TIME & DISTANCE | NOTES |
|---|---|---|
|  |  |  |
|  |  |  |
|  |  |  |
|  |  |  |
|  |  |  |

## ENVIRONMENT

| PLANTS |
|---|
|  |
| ANIMALS |
|  |

## ROUTE RATING

| DIFFICULTY | ☆☆☆☆☆ |
|---|---|
| ROAD CONDITION | ☆☆☆☆☆ |
| ENVIRONMENT | ☆☆☆☆☆ |

### ADDITIONAL NOTES

www.ingramcontent.com/pod-product-compliance
Lightning Source LLC
Chambersburg PA
CBHW081155070526
44583CB00021B/2848